POST-LINEAGE YOGA

POST-LINEAGE YOGA
From Guru to #MeToo

Theodora Wildcroft

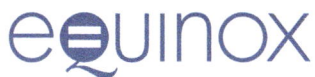

eQuinox

SHEFFIELD uk   BRISTOL ct

Published by Equinox Publishing Ltd.

UK: Office 415, The Workstation, 15 Paternoster Row, Sheffield,
South Yorkshire S1 2BX

USA: ISD, 70 Enterprise Drive, Bristol, CT 06010

www.equinoxpub.com

First published 2020

ISBN 978 1 78179 939 0 (hardback)
      978 1 78179 940 6 (paperback)
      978 1 78179 941 3 (ePDF)

British Library Cataloguing-in-Publication Data

A catalogue record for this book is available from the British Library.

Library of Congress Cataloging-in-Publication Data

Names: Wildcroft, Theodora, author.
Title: Post-lineage yoga : from guru to #metoo / Theodora Wildcroft, PhD.
Description: Sheffield, South Yorkshire ; Bristol, CT : Equinox Publishing Ltd, 2020. |
    Includes bibliographical references and index. | Summary: "This book presents a
    ground-breaking model for scholars to understand the contemporary teaching
    and practice of yoga"—Provided by publisher.
Identifiers: LCCN 2020020630 (print) | LCCN 2020020631 (ebook) |
    ISBN 9781781799390 (hardback) | ISBN 9781781799406 (paperback) |
    ISBN 9781781799413 (ePDF)
Subjects: LCSH: Hatha yoga—Study and teaching.
Classification: LCC RA781.7 .W54 2020 (print) | LCC RA781.7 (ebook) |
    DDC 613.7/046—dc23
LC record available at https://lccn.loc.gov/2020020630
LC ebook record available at https://lccn.loc.gov/2020020631

Typeset by JS Typesetting Ltd, Porthcawl, Mid Glamorgan

In memory of Collette, Matt and Gavin,
each lost too soon

CONTENTS

LIST OF FIGURES

PREFACE

This book addresses a significant lack in existing research into the lived experience of contemporary, transnational yoga practice. It starts from two premises: that what long-term practitioners are actually doing in their practice is important; and that the communities in which yoga is taught are vital sites for the production of subcultural knowledge. As a result, this book delivers a vivid portrait of an understudied subculture which little resembles the image of contemporary yoga held by yoga historians, debated by policy makers, and disseminated by mainstream media.

As I will show, post-lineage yoga may be uniquely developing as it comes into contact with a nature-focused British counterculture previously declared defunct. It is not high profile, and these practices, and their communities, are thus far invisible within media and scholarly accounts of transnational yoga. In fact, much of the rapidly evolving, diverse, and above all *moving* contemporary practice of yoga, involving hundreds of forms, schools and loose affiliations, is largely defined only by its perceived distance from the roots of what is often called 'traditional' yoga, and from traditional *guru-śiṣya* transmission (Burger 2006: 83). Herein, I address some of the reasons as to why such subcultures are so invisible within the wider culture and within academic understanding. Yoga scholars in particular do a great disservice to contemporary practitioners when we fail to take account of the true diversity, history, intention and experiences at the heart of contemporary yoga practice. In contrast, when we consider post-lineage yoga as that which moves beyond lineage as the sole authority for practice, we can discover much more about what is risked, gained and lost in this evolution.

Part I of this book sets out to define post-lineage yoga in detail. It begins with an introduction to the landscapes, people, and practices of a specific post-lineage yoga subculture, and how it compares with current academic and popular conceptions of contemporary yoga. Researching the specific subculture at the heart of this book necessitated the creation of an innovative methodology of co-practice, notation, and method as experiment that is newly fit for the purpose of studying bodily religious practice. In brief, that research method is detailed in Chapter 2, as a preliminary map for others to follow and expand. Chapter 3 explores a typical journey from the yoga mainstream to the spaces of post-lineage yoga, while Chapter

4 compares the cultural detail and ecology of three post-lineage yoga events: Colourfest, Santosa and Sundara.

This book compares individual practice with fieldwork at events where yoga teacher-practitioners alternate roles and inspire each other in unpredictable ways. Having provided a vivid portrait of post-lineage sub-culture, Part II of this book (Chapter 5) turns to a series of six, in-depth case studies of individual practitioners. These illustrate particular themes drawn from the fieldwork, and describe the intricate relationship between present practice and personal history.

Analysing this subculture further necessitated understanding the processes at the heart of practitioner negotiations with identity, ecology, and authority. That analysis gave rise to new models for understanding practice that were applicable to many more yogic subcultures than previously suspected. It also gave rise to the new term to describe them that is already being debated beyond the spaces of this research: post-lineage yoga. Part III of this book provides that analysis, linking personhood to practice, community to cultural repertoire. Chapter 6 details a model for understanding individual practice, while Chapters 7 and 8 explore the complex relationship between individual practice, teaching practice to others, and the creation of consensus repertoires of practice for the subculture. Chapter 9 brings the book full circle, connecting shared repertoires and shared experiences to community subcultures of the kind first introduced in Chapter 1.

In Chapter 10, the book concludes by extrapolating the models, processes and intentions at the heart of post-lineage yoga as part of a global revolution in how contemporary yoga is now taught. In 2004, Bikram Choudhury's global reach and his attempts to trademark a specific practice were held to be a prime example of dominant modern yoga brands (Carrette and King 2013: 8). In 2015, Choudhury's commercial empire collapsed, following his prosecution in absentia for sexual assault charges (Healy 2015). This collapse demonstrates how very different transnational yoga has become in the fifteen years since *Selling Spirituality* was published (Taylor 2018).

This book delivers therefore far more than a portrait of a fascinating subculture. It is representative of a rising trend: a questioning of established paradigms and authorities in yoga that will have profound and unforeseeable effects in the years to come. In this light, the attempts by Bikram Choudhury to apply copyright to this diverse, living practice could prove to have been the high watermark of decades of collaboration between modern lineage hierarchies and neoliberal business strategies (Puustinen and Rautaniemi 2015: 48).

While mindfulness apps and Instagram yoga stars are still in the business of selling yoga, we are also witnessing a widespread reckoning with abuses by high-profile teachers, and growing attempts to diversify the practice to marginalised and vulnerable populations. As I will show, all these developments are also characteristic of post-lineage yoga. Beyond the simple dichotomies of traditional versus commercial, spiritual versus secular, and indeed born of the productive tensions between them, post-lineage yoga defies easy categorisation.

ACKNOWLEDGEMENTS

Just as raising a child takes a village, writing this book took a saṃgha. There are too many people to name them all. But special thanks go to: Graham Harvey and Gwilym Beckerlegge for doctoral supervision above and beyond the call; to Mark Singleton, Suzanne Newcombe, Jason Birch and Jacqueline Hargreaves and the other scholars of the Hatha Yoga and AyurYoga Projects for friendship, mentoring and support; to Alison Robertson, David Robertson (no relation), Aled Thomas and the rest of the OU, BASR and RSP network, both early career and established academics, for inspirations, advice, collaborations and long conversations; and to Matthew Remski, Donna Farhi, Peter Blackaby and too many other yoga teachers and writers to mention, for being part of my own murmuration. And, of course, I give thanks to my editors and reviewers without whom this book would never have been published, and quite possibly still not have a proper title.

Above all, I thank my interviewees and my case studies, for their endless generosity, each and every one. I thank the Colourfest, Santosa, and Sundara saṃghas and so many other people I have spent sun-drenched, wind-swept, rain-washed days with, 'doing yoga in fields with hippies' as Graham puts it.

Finally, my unending love goes to my husband/handler Phil Wildcroft, who continues to provide caffeine regulation management and technical support.

आचार्यात् पादमादत्ते पादं शिष्यः स्वमेधया ।
पादं सब्रह्मचारिभ्यः पादं कालक्रमेण च ॥

ācāryāt pādamādatte pādaṃ śiṣyaḥ svamedhayā |
pādaṃ sabrahmacāribhyaḥ pādam kālakrameṇa ca ॥

A student receives a quarter [of knowledge] from the teacher, a quarter from his own intelligence, a quarter from fellow students and a quarter in the course of time.

– Traditional Sanskrit saying

PART I

DEFINING POST-LINEAGE YOGA

1
Introduction

In the shadow and stillness of a small and empty **yoga**[1] studio, a woman lights candles before stepping onto a mat and moving for almost an hour without stopping, drawing on practices from a dozen different teachers and the emergent desires of her body.

In a converted garage hung with hand-painted *yantras* (symbolic, geometric portraits of Hindu deities and other divine forms), another stretches out onto sheepskins and blankets, to the recorded sounds of a bubbling Irish spring.

Early one morning, another woman murmurs Sanskrit *mantras* (repetitive chanting with devotional or magical intent) in her kitchen, while she gathers supplies for her daily *pūjā* (devotional ritual consisting of chants and offerings made to figures on an altar).

And in the garden of a suburban home, a man bounces gently in and out of the deep press up position known as *caturaṅga daṇḍāsana*. He uses no yoga mat at all.

From London to Stroud to Bristol to the southern Welsh borders, each practice is as diverse as it is spontaneous, riding on the currents of memory, creative impulse and immediate need. But every so often, a shape or a posture or a way of breathing recurs, and the common culture that holds them becomes clear.

POST-LINEAGE YOGA IN CONTEXT

Millions of practitioners around the world today engage in a multitude of practices that they all call 'yoga'. This Sanskrit term covers a vast diversity of history and practice, philosophy and belief. Today, most people's

---

1 Terms in bold are included in the glossary.

mental image of modern yoga is of bodies moving and bodies sitting, in a practice for health and wellbeing that academics most often call 'modern postural yoga', after the ground breaking work of Elizabeth De Michelis (2007).

Yet in many contexts, in many cultural settings, yoga retains other meanings: as a metaphysical system describing the ongoing creation of the universe; as a devotional, ritual practice (Newcombe 2013: 72), and as a system of ethics and other social practices for righteous living. For the purposes of this book, we can cautiously define contemporary yoga as a practice of self-conscious, ritualised movement and stillness, focused on **somatic** or sensory experience, set within *subcultures* that are linked to diverse beliefs and engaged in complex relationships with the religions and cultures of the Indian sub-continent.

We can define a subculture as something larger than a community, yet smaller than a society. It denotes a grouping of people who are characterised by shared practices, activities, pastimes, lifestyles, art and other cultural reference points. Its membership is coherent and self-aware, and it exists in some way in both opposition to and relationship with the mainstream. A subculture describes both *things* (media and objects) and *people* (groups and communities).

The concept of subculture has a troubled academic history. Sociologists such as Dick Hebdige have neatly defined it as 'a form of refusal' expressed through styles of clothing and music (Hebdige 1979: 2). They place subcultures in absolute opposition to mainstream culture and consider them as an inevitable rebellious and youthful response to structural, societal changes such as were seen after the second world war. Later researchers have shifted to explore the practices, the self-understandings, and the diversity at the heart of lived subcultural experience. In my own research, I have also chosen to focus less on the cultural *products* of post-lineage yoga, and more on the *identities, communities* and *practices* involved. Each of those terms will receive much more attention in the course of this book.

As a result, my use of the term 'subcultures' here is a knowingly imperfect one, aimed at concentrating the reader's mind on what is fluid and what is fixed, what can be known and unknown. We are thus able to concentrate on the *processes* of negotiation at the heart of each participant's shifting allegiance to multiple and evolving group identity labels: that of yoga practitioner and teacher, lineage holder and activist, culture and subculture. So it is that the most relevant definition for a 'subculture' is that of Paul Sweetman, who uses it to describe:

relatively committed lifestyle groupings characterised by the gratuitous expenditure of energy on non-instrumental pleasures and 'extra-curricular' virtuosities, leading not only to the temporary appropriation of time and space, but the development of *alternative knowledges, capitals, bodies and subjectivities which may themselves stand apart from, or challenge, institutionalised or hegemonic forms.*

(Sweetman 2013: 7, emphasis added)

Given that definition, the most salient features of contemporary yoga are its diversity and rapid, ongoing evolution. This book takes just one community of yoga practice, but uses it in microcosm to represent a transnational revolution in how the practice is now performed, understood, and shared.

Among long-term yoga practitioners, there is growing awareness that practices considered to be 'traditional' are in many cases a modern invention, or at least, radical reinterpretations of older practices. The ethics and efficacy of modern postural yoga and its teachers are under growing scrutiny, and in some cases, even subject to legal action (Healy 2015). In part, this reflects increasing interest in some forms of yoga practice as an adjunct therapy for chronic health conditions, and thus a desire for such interventions to be as safe and predictable as possible. Nonetheless, dissatisfaction with modernised lineage models is mounting, as is criticism of standardised, commercial brands that are promoted using images of a largely unobtainable 'yoga body'. Heated debates about the 'authenticity' of specific practice forms, the extraction of wisdom techniques for commercial gain, and the 'true' meaning of the practice, often dominate the social media platforms, blogs, podcasts and articles of yoga-related media.

In this context, some communities, writers and teachers within contemporary yoga are evolving their relationships to the lineage and brand authorities under which they first dedicated themselves to a regular practice. To a lesser or greater extent, they are looking outside of these early sources of inspiration to determine what, for them, is labelled yoga. This is the under-researched phenomenon that I have labelled '**post-lineage yoga**'.

Post-lineage practitioners are radically altering the systems of transmission and authority that have previously been thought to define the boundaries of transnational yoga. And yet, post-lineage yoga is probably not an exclusively recent phenomenon. Terms such as lineage and brand, modern postural and post-lineage, describe forces that unevenly shape subcultures along a continuum. What is often considered to be traditional, lineage-based yoga, is also a departure from the past, evolving in response to the forces of modernity. It may be that not only is post-lineage yoga a more *common* phenomenon than it first appears, but also that it might be more *historically distributed* than current research can account for. Beyond the practice sanctioned by major lineages, ashrams and historical texts, as historians of yoga seek to understand the vernacular precedents and historical authority structures of postural practice (Broo 2015), there may be a very different picture to emerge. What we can be sure of, is the growing self-awareness, interpersonal networking, and visibility of grassroots, non-institutional forms of yoga transmission in the Anglophone world, for over a decade or more.

Previous to this, more easily identifiable, more well-known and more self-contained systems of yoga rose to prominence partly as a result of nineteenth-century encounters between India, Europe and America, mediated by orientalist ideas, and partly in response to the Indian independence movement and a postcolonial revival in Indian physical culture (Singleton 2013: 39). Both emic and etic commentaries on yoga still use these prominent lineages as shorthand for both authentic and standard practice to this day. Furthermore, sociological research into contemporary yoga largely investigates only its most ubiquitous and commercially successful expressions, and its most casual practitioners, who attend a weekly class mostly for general physical wellbeing and social interaction. In comparison to such a narrow if numerous population, the events and people profiled in this book will appear unusually dedicated, even obsessively reflexive about the practice of yoga. My respondents are people who have devoted many years, and countless hours, not only to post-lineage practice, but to understanding what it means to them. At some events, as many as 80 per cent are also yoga teachers, many of them teaching as their primary professional identity.

The conclusion of many academics, as demonstrated in Carrette and King (2013) and challenged by Jain (2014a), is that modern yoga *practitioners* have little more than a shallow comprehension of their own practice. But in fact, for transnational yoga, claims to historical precedence, metaphysical and scientific epistemologies, and the ethics of its most well-known teaching structures are all being tested on an unprecedented scale, and far from remaining ignorant of this process, informal yoga *teacher* networks are evolving in response.

To give just two examples, Mark Singleton's 2010 book, *Yoga Body*, had a seismic impact on transnational yoga. Now widely read and debated in

English-speaking yoga subcultures, its main focus is the socio-cultural background and motivations of the originators of early modern yoga: Krishnamacharya, BKS Iyengar, Swami Sivananda, Pattabhi Jois, and other, less well-known teachers. In the first half of the twentieth-century, they and their counterparts reclaimed the indigenous practice of **haṭhayoga**[2] from its decadent associations and reformed it with reference to such diverse sources as the YMCA, Nature Cure, therapeutic gymnastics, calisthenics and body building. Adding to this picture, a less well known body of work by Joseph Alter (2005, 2006, 2012) describes the processes by which the practices thus recovered or discovered were wedded to claims of ancient Hindu authenticity in the service of Indian independence and postcolonial nationalism.

More recently, Singleton co-authored with James Mallinson a second key historical text: *Roots of Yoga* (Mallinson and Singleton 2017). This attempts to make sense for the reader of a breath-taking diversity of pre-modern source texts, dividing them into categories familiar to any serious yoga student, such as Posture, Breath-control and the Yogic Body. It provides even more context for understanding the extent to which contemporary yoga is both a continuation with, and departure from, its historical antecedents. With the release of *Yoga Body* and *Roots of Yoga*, we are starting to see the persistent myth of 'traditional yoga' as a singular, coherent and primordially authentic practice form come to an end.

Both books are already established within the Yoga Studies academic canon. But scholars may not realise that they are also now included on numerous yoga teacher training syllabi. These books join an increasing number of texts and courses aimed at yoga teachers and practitioners which tackle different aspects of yoga history and present the latest yoga-related scientific research. Together they reveal to teacher-practitioners themselves that the roots of this transnational practice are diverse, fragmented and heavily blended, and its effects on its practitioners are equally diverse, complex, and contingent on circumstance. While yoga practitioners may differ on the validity they accord to such research as it emerges, few yoga teachers are ignorant of the debates it is provoking, and some are re-narrating their own yoga origin stories in response. Acknowledging that what is considered to be traditional practice might involve significant

---

2 A collection of practices that traditionally includes *āsana*, *prāṇāyāma* and meditation, for much of its history associated with certain anti-social behaviours, reclaimed as the foundation of modern postural yoga.

innovation in the modern era has led to a wider 'hunger in the yoga community for writing about yoga that is critical, challenging, political, and relevant to life in the 21st century' (Horton and Harvey 2012: 181).

The complex cross-fertilisation of scholarly and practitioner, scientific and cultural theories in fact has a long history within communities of dedicated yoga practitioners, even if this is not a discourse found within the average drop-in yoga class. The common mistake made by researchers thus far is in assuming that the teacher and long-term residents of such classes are unaware of that discourse as the larger context for what is being taught. 'Yoga reoriented is new theory with old practice' (Singleton and Byrne 2008: 71). But modern yoga is also arguably new practice with radical reinterpretations of even older theory. Within the neo-Vedāntic modernist yoga renaissance (Singleton 2013: 38), echoes of the medieval Tantric roots of *haṭhayoga* as counter-caste, embodied alchemy are retained and can be seen in a number of texts by contemporary practitioners, including books authored by two of my case studies: Dinsmore-Tuli (2013b) and Gladwell and Wender (2014).

SOME MOTIVATIONS FOR EXPLORING BEYOND LINEAGE

My research suggests that in Britain at least, post-lineage yoga practitioners tend to be countercultural, highly educated, ecological, inspired by the complex interplay of Hindu, New Age and European holism, and concerned with the innovative, the obscure, and with how the practice promotes social justice. Above all, they are not casual consumers of a practice led by spiritual entrepreneurs. Many teach, some write, others are highly respected among their peers, and these may influence the lived experiences of far more practitioners of yoga than suspected.

In recent history, this heritage of little-known radical yoga practitioners includes such people as Angela Farmer. Angela was one of the earliest and most senior teachers to publicly distance themselves from the **Iyengar Yoga** system: a well-known *āsana*-based[3] practice for health that very closely follows the original teachings of BKS Iyengar. She went on to become one of the most influential yoga teachers of what is often labelled the '**divine feminine**'[4] school of practice. She even invented the modern

---

3 Involving physical poses and movement.
4 A school of feminist religious thought, with associated yoga forms that focus on female representation and practices appropriate for female bodies.

yoga mat (Ruiz 2007). She still runs workshops and retreats, together with her partner, Victor van Kooten, and between them they have over a century of experience teaching yoga. And yet, to date, the only significant profile of her is one, obscure film (Cummins 1997). Otherwise, her story, and the stories of most significant yoga figures working outside of lineage hierarchies, remains largely untold.

A significant number of my respondents, like Angela and Victor, have weathered some form of loss of trust in the lineages that trained them. Credible evidence continues to emerge of misconduct, criminality, and serious interpersonal abuse, by a significant number of the modern gurus and senior teachers of yoga, from the lurid details of Geoffrey Falk's *Stripping the Gurus* (2009), to Matthew Remski's case study of a lineage hierarchy perpetuating and justifying the persistent sexual assault committed by its founder (Remski 2019). McKean (1996) is just one example of a number of texts examining the social and political power wielded within the guru system (see also Storr 1997; Kramer and Alstad 2012). And for Singleton and Goldberg, 'The rejection of gurus' authority on moral and rational grounds [...] has a strong history within modern India' (2013a: 8). And yet other commentaries on the development of modern yoga practice are often silent on the troubled history of the guru system.

More common are calls for yogic transmission to more closely model traditional discipleship, and in so doing anchor yoga to its 'original' purpose, such as in Liberman (2008) and Burger (2006). Many, like Maya Burger (2006), place the blame for abuse by gurus on yoga's reception in Anglo-American and European culture, with little critical analysis of any role gurus might play themselves in this process. In contrast, it can be persuasively argued that outside of yoga's indigenous context, assumptions that gurus are ethically faultless created the very cover under which many such abuses flourished with impunity.

To retrofit pre-modern transmission relationships to the modern era, as I will show, is to muddle the intent of practice with its teaching style, and the teacher's level of spiritual liberation with their charisma. It is also profoundly elitist: confining the *history* of yoga to its most privileged teachers, and the *present and future* of 'authentic' yoga to its more affluent, educated practitioners. There is no self-evident connection between an individual's level of spiritual attainment, and their ability to transmit the same realisations to a congregation of hundreds, thousands, or more, by means of teaching modern postural yoga. And what is reframed in this concept of the corrupted Eastern ascetic is often the long-term sexual and spiritual abuse of (mostly female) disciples and their children by (mostly male) authority figures who claimed unerring moral purity and absolute power over their followers' daily living and spiritual development through infinite reincarnations. These are not minor social transgressions in the face of unaccustomed temptation (Remski 2014a).

Neither the detail of guru scandals and the ways in which lineage is structured to protect power, nor the complex entanglements of race, gender, colonialism and religion are the main focus of this book. Yet these ethical failures show that detailing methods of transmission and patterns of authority are more than an academic exercise. At stake is the wellbeing and self-determination of millions of practitioners, and the postcolonial evolution of a vast and diverse Indian cultural phenomenon.

As I will show, embracing post-lineage sources of authority is only a practitioner's first step in negotiating power, charisma and privilege in teaching and in practice. The formal and implicit hierarchies of multiple schools of yoga collide in every post-lineage subcultural landscape. Each teacher and practitioner must hold the others to account, creating shifting patterns of recommendations, professional alliances, and more intimate connections with their peers. Other forms of personal capital tip the scales of social standing: how adaptable a teacher is, how rooted their lives are in practices of advocacy and activism, and how familiar they are with the tropes of social justice, and established countercultural norms. The evolving consensus of a post-lineage yoga subculture is contested and renewed at every communal event, with every self-published guide to practice, in every travelling teacher's workshop, and, indeed, every time each practitioner steps on a yoga mat.

This book explores one such post-lineage subculture, at the heart of which are a number of modern yoga practitioners who came together in some way dissatisfied with their existing experience of yoga. Some had injured themselves doing practices they had been taught were universally safe. Some had enjoyed practices that felt liberational, and then discovered patriarchal abuses within the schools that taught them. In a number of cases, these negative experiences compounded issues that brought them to yoga practice in the first place. Modern postural and post-lineage yoga are both methods of incremental transformation. By definition, more devoted practitioners often find their initial dedication to regular practice in the changes they want to make in themselves. Anecdotally, these commonly involve lingering lower back pain, general anxiety, and the many other chronic conditions that mainstream medical practice has less success in managing: such as fibromyalgia or complex PTSD. Yoga is a health-forwarding activity. But in the end, and as my case studies will demonstrate, some practitioners pass for healthy precisely because their suffering and their healing is contained within the practice.

When the existing practice or communities of modern postural yoga no longer served their needs, however, these post-lineage practitioners did not walk away from yoga entirely. Instead, they came together, finding in group solidarity a new way to practise, and joined by those whose schools of yoga were more open to inter-lineage exchanges of knowledge and fellowship. While individual practitioners may or may not maintain close connections to their original teachers, post-lineage subcultures have a common and definitional relationship to the established authorities of modern yoga. They reject the idea that any individual yogic text or modern alignment paradigm can hold complete universal truth, and reject unquestioning allegiance to a single deity in the form of a living or historical figure. They reject the still-common practice of attributing any harm caused within the practice to defects in the practitioner, and seek to re-situate the practice in community, and socio-political contexts. Post-lineage yoga is, at heart, a re-evaluation of the authority to determine practice, and a privileging of peer networks over pedagogical hierarchies, or *saṃgha*s (communities) over *guru-śiṣya* (teacher-adept) relationships.

At the **Santosa** event, in 2016, I was invited to chair a wide flowing, passionate discussion about what might be meant by the term 'post-lineage yoga'. Most participants in the discussion had already been wrestling for some time with the question of authority over practice. All were anxious to honour the immense gifts that their lineage-based trainings continued to confer on their practice. But all of them found support for the *ongoing* evolution of that practice in communities where practitioners from many lineages and none came together. Some talked about the death of a beloved teacher. Others discussed ethical failures within specific lineage communities. Many talked about broadening their knowledge, and being more comfortable within peer-based authority structures. All of them continued to debate the risks and rewards of moving from lineage to peer-based communities of knowledge.

During the discussion, some practitioners described issues with networking with the more dogmatic and isolationist lineages, or schools with very vertical hierarchies. I asked if any teacher had ever taught at Santosa who was still officially affiliated to the British Iyengar Yoga organisation. I was told that an affiliated teacher had taught at Santosa just once, but the national lineage leadership had to be consulted, and stipulated that the event could not be advertised on any of their forums, as non-Iyengar Yoga teachers would also be teaching. One person there even said: 'The Iyengar police are real.'

This level of debate among yoga teachers and long-term practitioners is not unique to the spaces of my research. Yoga as an endeavour is often framed as an individual journey, undertaken through personal practice, in the search for inner wisdom. Familiar from both historical tradition (Mallinson and Singleton 2017: 52) and the narrow representations of yoga in mass marketing, each yoga practice is a reproducible but individual experience, contained by the existential island that is each person's yoga mat. But at its most contemplative or its most standardised, contemporary yoga is likely to involve significant periods of direct teaching, body to body, person to person. Similarly, post-lineage yoga arises in a specifically negotiated relationship between individual exploration and various forms of group sharing. As we will see, the patterns of authority that govern this relationship include three sources: the internal wisdom of the self, the external authority of the expert, and the relational opinion of the group. Consciously or not, each change in practice or ethics is justified by one or more of these. The one most often absent from most discussions of yogic authority, in scholarship or in cultural discourse, is the latter, the group.

A FIRST PORTRAIT OF A POST-LINEAGE SUBCULTURE

As a number of commentators have stated, the semiotics of transnational yoga brands and global meditational schools are employed to market health-related products from corporate mindfulness to diet food (Carrette and King 2013: 16; Sanders and Mouyis 2010). But there is a clear and stark difference between yoga imagery as conceived by marketing executives and used to sell yoghurt, and yoga as a living religious practice. As post-lineage yoga is an understudied, but also material and lived practice, my most urgent task is to introduce the unique character of the people and places of my research: through the shared subculture of three post-lineage yoga events, spanning the British summer, from **Colourfest** in June, to **Sundara** in July, and Santosa in August.

Let us begin with that yoga mat. As both place and symbol of one's investment in the practice it is freighted with personal history in the abstract and specific. And fittingly for an individualised and idiosyncratic subculture, each group session here is a mosaic of mats of all qualities and materials, including sheepskins, blankets, or no mat at all, laid out on the dusty grass or under the dripping canvas of practice spaces. Clothing is a more reliable indicator of one's membership of smaller affinity groups, and different clothes enhance specific experiences. In more energetic sessions, clothing is often minimal, and as taut and flexible as its practitioners. Adepts of practices described as 'soft' or more fluid are more likely to wear softer fabrics and more flowing lines. Those whose practices have soteriological aims are more likely to wear white and purple. Those whose aims are more earth-bound wear more greens, reds, and earthy tones. Many wear second hand, eclectically patterned and homemade clothes.

Like many religious communities food is important to this subculture (Harvey 2014: 29–30), both in what is eaten and the rituals that surround it. It is always vegetarian, and communal food is often vegan. Everything on offer fits shifting definitions of 'sattvic' or holistically balancing food, and a high proportion is organic. This subculture associates such food with nourishment, while the food produced by corporate agribusiness, like much of modern life, is seen as polluting.

Purifying and cleansing practices are a central feature of all these events, consistent with numerous traditional *haṭhayoga* practices such as

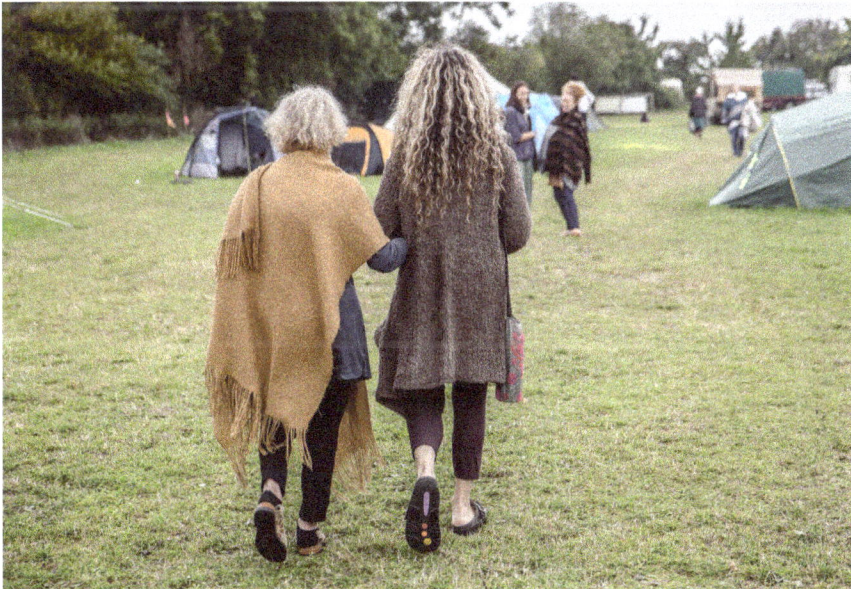

Figure 1.1
Santosa: Walking with friends (photograph by Letitia Valverdes)

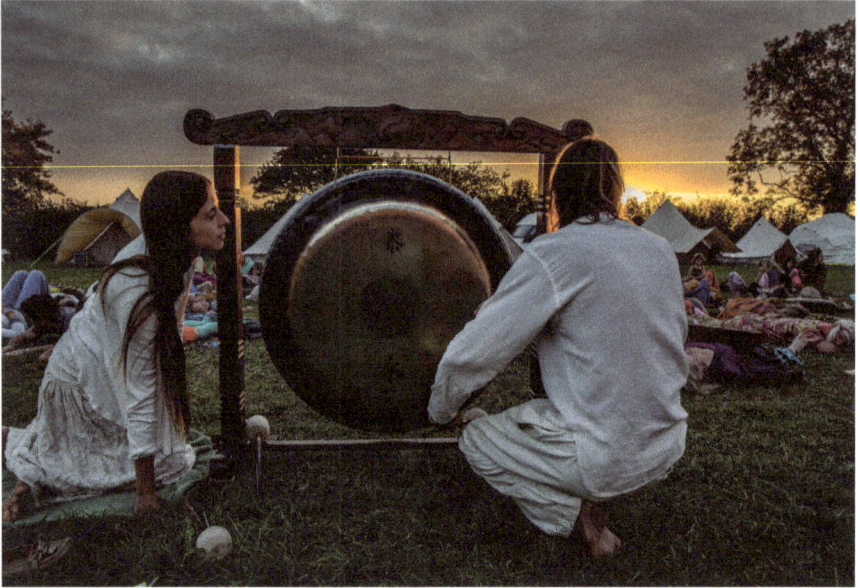

Figure 1.2

Santosa: Playing gongs during a ceremony (photograph by Letitia Valverdes)

ṣaṭkarman (Birch 2011: 3). Many sites feature well-attended saunas. Burning sage, mugwort or Palo Santo are also used to purify spaces and participants; fire and water being seen as the most transformative elements.

Traditional Hindu prohibitions concerning the unclean status of certain individuals, specifically menstruating women, are completely absent, although some practices are commonly contraindicated as being less 'nourishing' for pregnant, menstruating, or breastfeeding women. In their place are prohibitions on both legal and illegal intoxicant use, although certain mildly entheogenic plants, including mugwort and cacao, are embraced within specific consciousness-altering practices. These events, like the emerging phenomenon of yoga raves, supplement a solitary practice experience with an added relational dimension (Jacobs 2017: 2). But while participants in a rave commonly encounter ecstatic experiences of 'communality, equality and basic humanity' (Olaveson 2004: 87), these events are characterised by experiences that are closer to that which Judith Kovach (2002: 949) describes as enstatic experiences, without a hedonistic loss of control or responsibility.

George Lakoff and Mark Johnson argue that bodies, minds and ecologies are inseparable, and that an embodied spirituality is necessarily an ethical orientation to the land (Lakoff and Johnson 1999: 566). Fittingly, the ecology of post-lineage yoga is a fundamental aspect of the practice. My participants come to their yoga mats, alone or together, in new ways of being, relating, and understanding. These events are thus spaces in which to practise a different relationship to the land, idealised and aspirational but also pragmatic. Participants are encouraged to engage with their environment in various devotional acts. Within many taught sessions, affirmations to attune to 'higher vibrations' alternate with instructions to 'ground' and 'arrive' and honour the immediate ecology. Balanced between land and sky, earth and heaven, each group session involves participants coming together:

> [in] this simple life, where miracles are the essence of every stitch in the tapestry of time and feeling, and arms unfold across worlds.
>
> (Dance Jam session, Colourfest)

The practice is as diverse here as the environment: movements and postures have less precision, fewer straight lines, and more individuality than the average yoga class. Contemplation is less about withdrawing from the world, and more about sitting in easeful relationship with the weather, the uneven ground, and the sounds of other activities. This sense of the sacredness of physical existence extends beyond place to those natural miracles of living existence usually considered to be mundane, from menstruation to evolution. In one **Scaravelli Inspired Yoga**[5] session at Colourfest, we are told:

> There was a tail there once upon a time. [...] See if you can sense that sense of maybe awakening the sacrum, the lower back. And then what you can do if you like is just put your hand on your lower back, like you've got a tail here now, and give it a little wiggle.

Every religious practice adapts to the 'qualities and physical expressions' of the places in which they take place, becoming unavoidably vernacular in the process (Whitehead 2008: 167). Tantric or Ayurvedic metaphysics of the five elements or qualities of matter: earth, water, fire, air and

---

5 There is a loose school of 'divine feminine' yoga practices inspired by the lifework of Vanda Scaravelli, who asked her students not to name a school after her. 'Scaravelli Inspired' is a self-chosen label that expresses a teacher's compromise between honouring that request and the need to signal the kind of approach they use in teaching.

ākāśa (variously translated as spirit, ether and space) are commonly used as teaching metaphors here. But they intersect with neopagan understandings of the immediate ritual ecology of four directions, in their correspondences to earth, air, fire and water, temporally expressed through the waxing and waning of the Wheel of the Year (Whitehead 2008: 171). These elements wax and wane in human bodies too. The concepts associated with such elemental and internal energies thus refer interchangeably to somatic experiences, frequencies of matter, personality characteristics, and metaphors for tension and change.

The detail of these qualities and their correspondences may vary, but their overall alignment renders possible the translation of sub-tropical non-dual ritual practices into a temperate British ecology. While the people, places and practices thus become mutable and permeable (Johnson 2002: 314), they are not, however, rendered placeless as a result. They are instead subject to the contrasting processes of what Thomas Tweed calls 'dwelling' and 'crossing' (Tweed 2006).

COMPARING POST-LINEAGE YOGA WITH THE VISIBLE YOGA MAINSTREAM

How different, therefore, is the yoga that is at the heart of this research from the aforementioned widely recognised forms of yoga? Despite the diversity of schools and lineages, a broad sketch of a typical modern postural yoga lesson is commonly recognisable. It occurs in a clean, tidy space, with identical, teacher-provided mats carefully aligned and the teacher's place and role distinct from that of students. The practice itself is conceived of as a series of set physical positions, with clear transitions, and a more or less universalised alignment of process and posture. It conforms closely to the practice learnt by the teacher during their own teacher training. In Britain at least, that training was in one of the dominant lineages or schools of Iyengar, **Ashtanga**,[6] or **Sivananda Yoga**,[7] or in a more generic studio setting, often labelled **Hatha Yoga**,[8] and accredited by **Yoga Alliance Professionals** (no relation to **Yoga Alliance**, based in

---

6 A specific *āsana* and *vinyāsa* based practice fixed during the modern Mysore yoga revival by Pattabhi Jois.

7 Patañjali-inspired yoga practice developed from the teachings of Swami Sivananda.

8 This designation is often used when a contemporary yoga practice is outside the most common and visible lineages, or used to designate a gentler practice form.

the US), or the **British Wheel of Yoga**. It might even be one of the much less intensive trainings in the basic postures of yoga accredited for fitness instructors. It will appear to be focused on health and wellbeing, and thus broadly secular, although more esoteric, axiological and philosophical content will be evident from closer examination. This sequence is typical of the instruction in many classes:

> *Hanumanasana.* This challenging yet graceful posture [...] refers to the fantastic leaps this popular deity took in service to his master Rama. [...] Once the legs are straight, sit on the floor and bring the hands together in a prayer position in front of the chest [...] Stay in this position for ten breaths or more.
>
> (Brown 2009: 166–7)

When the NHS recommends yoga as a gentle form of exercise appropriate to the masses, it has a specific idea of what that yoga should look like (see NHS Fitness Studio 2016). It might not have the fast paced athleticism and commercial innovation of recent transatlantic yoga brands such as Jivamukti Yoga (see https://jivamuktiyoga.com), which are as yet mostly confined to a few major UK cities. Its norms arise from a number of historical collaborations between local authorities, the Iyengar Yoga lineage and the British Wheel of Yoga (Hasselle-Newcombe 2005: 305–6), all of which have episodically attempted to systematise the transmission of yoga in Britain into a unified, safe, 'spiritual but not religious' system (Newcombe 2013: 68; Pettit 2014: 13). Recent responses by the wider British yoga community to the proposal of optional National Occupational Standards for yoga prove how contested that aim is (see Yoga Alliance UK 2016; Yates 2016; Remski 2016a). This reflects the increasingly obvious fact that the vast majority of less commercially oriented and less culturally dominant contemporary yoga subcultures are as yet invisible to policy makers and bureaucratic institutions.

The yoga in this book has significant differences from the standardised, branded practice characteristic of the most visible and dominant schools. It takes place in spaces with soft edges and unclear boundaries, where the ecology, weather, and other people can intrude. In its taught sessions, teachers take turns to step into the role. Practitioners experiment with multiple forms, without demonstrating a commitment to a single teacher. The teachers themselves most often hold allegiance to either a little-known lineage or none at all, and are often members of smaller organisations such as the **Independent Yoga Network**. They were usually first trained by a dominant lineage or generic organisation, but now look beyond that training to evolve both their individual and teaching practice.

At one five-day camp in 2016, there was not a single session labelled with a major lineage. In such contexts, the practice is more unpredictable, and experimental, and diversity, self-reliance and free movement are emphasised. The following instructions from a Yoga and Sounds session at Colourfest are typical:

> Next time you come up into down dog let's stay a little while. Keep it moving, so bend one knee then the other, then both knees together, or high up on to the toes. [...] Whatever feels good. Come out of the pose if you feel you need to. Be intuitive.

The image of contemporary yoga as it is understood by large brands, public policy and much academic scholarship, contrasts strongly with these environments. And yet again, post-lineage yoga may be much more prevalent than its lack of visibility suggests. It may be that the reality of contemporary yoga as taught in community halls and gyms across the world, and specifically as practised by yoga teachers themselves, is more democratic, devotional and idiosyncratic than we yet know.

The three events at the heart of my research are however specifically influenced by a long-standing tradition of outdoor festival events in Britain, from raucous May fairs (Walford 1878: 345) to Stonehenge jazz camps (Worthington 2004: 23). These are popularly associated with countercultural hedonism, temporary autonomy and community experiences of enchantment common to bioregional ecology movements (Baker 2015; Partridge 2005: 21). Like other such countercultural events, these camps are small in scale and little-known, and this can be deliberate. They are spaces to retreat, regroup, and refuel:

> I think gatherings and camps will always be a part of human life and if that stopped, I think there would be a big degradation in society.
>
> (John, co-organiser of Sundara)

These events find their niche between civilisation and the wild, more or less consciously echoing Henri David Thoreau's ideal dwelling position, halfway between woods and village (Gura 2006: 134–5). Thoreau referred to himself as a *yogī* (Broad 2012: 22), and by the turn of the twentieth century, his work had more influence in Britain than on his native America

(Harding 2006: 7). By the 1970s, the rise of the environmental movement that took Thoreau as one of its leading inspirations (Harding 2006: 10) was accompanied by an emerging counterculture that widely embraced yoga and meditation.

Thus overlapping generations of British counterculture collaborate at the heart of this particular yoga subculture: those who dropped out to create the early music festival scene (Moberg and Ramstedt 2016: 159) and the protest community from Greenham Common; travellers from the Stonehenge Peace Convoy and settlers from Tipi Valley; Newbury road protestors and people who ran sound systems at M25 raves and Welsh free parties; and now activists from climate camps, Occupy and the Calais Jungle.

But in other ways, they have less in common with the 'heroic ethics' of environmental protest activism (Gaard 2001: 14), and more to do with every-day acts of right relationship. Cleaning the toilets at Santosa is described as 'the highest *sadhana*', a word that encompasses ego-transcending spiritual practices, here adapted to the ideals of ecofeminism and bioregionalism (Gaard 2010: 653). Ethical norms here are influenced by Mahatma Gandhi's teachings on becoming a good citizen through service, justice, and moderating one's consumption habits (Godrej 2012: 450).

Above all, this is a subculture coming to terms with its own disillusion-ment with the endless health and abundance promised by yoga gurus, institutions and brands alike. In this it forms part of a growing 'culture of descent' (Dark Mountain Project 2010: 4) beginning to tell the stories that lie beyond the peak of late capitalism. It resituates the discourse of yoga practice, away from promises of unending positive progress (Langølen 2012: 36; Smith 2008: 147), and closer to rhythms of cyclical transforma-tion inspired by both Hinduism and modern paganism. As **Uma**, the sub-ject of Case study 3 and founder of Santosa explained:

> I think it promotes a real respect and gratitude. And out of that also a recon-nection that we are nothing but earth, you know?

Each individual finds their own way to relate to the post-lineage network in practice, affinity, authority and knowledge. As I will show, the subcul-ture evolves at least in part through a series of revelations and disillusion-ments, each shared by a few and supported by the many. Inevitably some leave the networks entirely, and some find other, hopefully more reliable or at least relatable teachers:

When **Babaji**[9] came into my life there was a card, I picked a card of his sayings and the card was 'be ordinary' and I really loved that.

(Trishula, organiser of the Beltane Bhakti Gathering)

DEBATES CONCERNING AUTHENTICITY AND RADICALISM

In the course of my research, some respondents used the term 'radical' to describe this subculture. While it implies both innovation and transformation, 'radical' is always a relational term, whose meaning is inferred from its conventional opposite. Etymologically, it also contains a sense of the foundational, or rooted. As is common within religious movements, yoga hagiographies and new commentaries on ancient texts continually reframe and (re)invent traditional narratives (Glassie 1995: 399) to redraw the foundations of the practice. In this way, associations with tradition are used to confer a sense of authenticity to practices that may be considered to be radical in other ways.

This book does not seek to pass judgement on the merit of claims of authenticity. That is a task more suited to theology or historical studies than contemporary ethnography. Luckily a focus on more unusual and idiosyncratic yoga subcultures affords me the welcome possibility of escaping the dominant debates about which revered gurus, and thus which lineages and practices, are more authentic than others (Satlow 2011: 135, in Newcombe 2016). It is much more productive here to consider authenticity as a quality that both confers and recognises asymmetries of power within interpersonal relationships (Pratt 1992: 7 in Kraft 2002: 162). Yoga practice is both holistic in its sphere of effect, and highly interoceptive in its results. The association of even the most physical forms of practice with psychological and spiritual benefit renders its mastery to an extent unfalsifiable. Put simply, *enlightenment can only be recognised by those who have achieved it*. As a result, the categories of 'true' and 'false' teacher of yoga are endlessly contested.

Nonetheless, my starting hypothesis is that British post-lineage teacher-practitioners sit, often consciously, within an ideological heritage of nature-honouring, materially embodied practitioners engaged in the pursuit of social justice. This heritage can itself be the source for a similar precedent-related authenticity to that afforded by more formal lineages

---

9 Sri Haidakhandi Babaji: one of numerous Hindu saints known as Babaji.

(for examples see Dinsmore-Tuli and Harrison 2015; Walker 2012). A long legacy of such teachers and writers inspired and continue to inspire each other as well as diverse practice communities. They can be considered a shared heritage, and in some cases even a religious 'chain of memory' (Hervieu-Léger 2000: 123). In the specific case of British contemporary post-lineage subcultures, such a chain would include W. B. Yeats (1938) and Aleister Crowley, who authored 'a textbook on the eight-step yoga path [...] in 1913' (Melton 1990: 503, in Singleton 2010: 66). It would include key female figures such as Indra Devi and Annie Besant (Goldberg 2016b), Sister Nivedita (Reymond 1985), and more recent figures such as Vanda Scaravelli (1991). This heritage forms a coherent chain of ideas that has been a significant source of inspiration within countercultural yoga subcultures for well over a century, from the beginnings of Theosophy onward (Chryssides 2012: 249). As Walter Harding reminds us:

> When Gandhi later settled in South Africa to give legal aid to Indian laborers suffering under segregation laws, he adopted Thoreau's *On the Duty of Civil Disobedience* as a manual of arms in his nonviolent fight for freedom.
> (Harding 2006: 7)

A number of my research participants referenced the life stories, poetry and wisdom of such radical figures as Mahatma Gandhi, Lalla Ded (Ded and Hoskote 2013), and above all Henry David Thoreau, as often as they did the traditional yoga citations from Patañjali's *Yogasūtra* or the *Bhagavad Gītā*. Just as post-lineage yoga is an understudied contemporary phenomenon, the wealth of historical literature it inherits is less evident within the academic record of yoga. Notable exceptions include work by Suzanne Newcombe (2013) on the early modern cross-fertilisation between yoga and the European occult. And Hugh Urban (2004) connects neopagan and New Age reimaginings of Tantric practices to a long history of occult interest in yoga. However, between the Tantric Sex websites and online Sanskrit seminars on Kashmir Shaivism that Urban takes as his sources, there is a world of nuance that he often elides. Once again, there is a tendency on the part of scholars to take more superficial examples of contemporary yoga as representative of the whole.

Many of my respondents, like Thoreau, are lay researchers of ancient yoga-related texts, albeit most often in translation. They, like he, take radical inspiration from yogic philosophy and practice, while rejecting the more prescriptive aspects of yogic institutions. Thoreau's own physical practice consisted of simply walking, and he wrote: 'We need pray for no higher heaven than the pure senses can furnish, a purely sensuous life' (Thoreau 2003). As Charlene Spretnak writes:

> the Levelers, Diggers, Muggletonians, Familists, Behmenists, Fifth Monarchy Men, Ranters, and Seekers were [also] associated with beliefs that God is present in everything in nature (panentheism), that matter is alive, that change occurs through internal dynamics rather than a rearrangement of parts, and that any individual can have direct experience of the divine.
>
> (Spretnak 2012: 133)

Throughout history, countercultural moments of resistance to 'the mechanistic, atomistic worldview of modernity' (Spretnak 2012: 133) recur again and again, sharing a framework of values based on ecological, spiritual, material, and bodily concerns, negotiated as human and more than human commons. The work of Matthew Remski (2015c), Uma Dinsmore-Tuli (2013b; see also Glossary), and many other post-lineage yoga practitioner-scholars, is often written as explicit political and social commentary. To this day, when radical reform movements seek practices and inspirations to build a capacity for awe, resilience and hope, they, like Gandhi and Thoreau, often turn to yoga and meditation (for examples see Rowe 2015; White 2016).

In very generalised terms, the modern postural yoga renaissance adapted the self-mortifying asceticism and supernatural rewards of medieval *haṭhayoga* in the service of purifying the mind, body and spirit for social harmony and divine and material reward. But in the textual record there exists evidence of an alternative history, in which yoga philosophy and practice appears to be employed by some, at various points in time, as a practice of re-embodiment for political and social reform, and personal healing and reconciliation with the natural world.

Matthew Remski (2014d) claims we are now seeing the end of the modernist yoga project that Elizabeth De Michelis's categorisation and Mark Singleton's historical analysis so beautifully delineates, with the recent deaths of its last gurus, and the rising reclamation of yoga by its practitioners, especially women. In considering only the most visible incarnations of contemporary yoga, we have been in fact, ignoring a long and storied heritage of re-enchanting bodies through unorthodox, community-based forms of post-lineage yoga, as a form of resistance to modernity and commercialisation. This is the context, the inspiration and the fuel for the untold story that this book seeks to tell.

2
Researching post-lineage yoga

Researching the specific subculture at the heart of this book necessitated the creation of an innovative methodology of co-practice, notation, and method as experiment that is newly fit for the purpose of studying bodily religious practice. In brief, that research method and the reasoning that supports it is detailed here, as a preliminary map for others to follow and expand.

But this chapter offers more than just a novel method for research. It includes a full description of the notation system used throughout the book, as a codex for the reader to unlock a much fuller understanding of the practice under consideration. And as I will show, in certain key ways, *researching* post-lineage yoga in this way reproduces and thus illuminates a number of the fault lines, slippages and unforeseen opportunities of *teaching* post-lineage yoga, that in turn fuel the ongoing evolution of shared cultures and shared repertoires at the heart of the practice.

Under consideration is not yoga as it is currently understood by wider contemporary culture, but as it is lived and practised by those most invested in that ongoing evolution. My participants are part of a loose network of people, the majority of whom consider yoga to be part of their personal and professional identity. They share significant experiences of disillusionment with mainstream yoga, and choose to respond by coming together in non-commercial, non-institutional spaces to share yoga practice. Other similar events exist. But these events in particular involve a weight of history and a coherent community of people, and as a result are clearly a significant vector for post-lineage yoga transmission here in the UK. My aim was clear: to explore their lived experience of the practice, the intentions informing that practice, and the subculture that supports it.

I had not begun with a theory to be tested, but rather an anomaly to be investigated. What followed, then, was a personal exploration of *method as experimentation*, developing a multi-layered process in which at each point the embodied understanding of both myself and participants was tested for its ability to produce useful and robust data (Wacquant 2014: 4).

Mine is a mixed methodology of linked processes: fieldwork and participation in both personal and taught practices, recordings of the same, and finally, interviews about both individual practices, and group environments. In order to enable comparison between specific individual practices, professional identities and sub-cultural processes, these different methods involved the same community, and in many cases, the same respondents. Each medium can be seen as a different lens that produces diverse data with an overlapping but non-identical scope. As the research progressed, the slippage between experience, observation, narration and transmission of practice became a way to understand some of the processes of sub-cultural evolution itself.

THE ACADEMIC BODY, THE EXPERT BODY, AND POSITIONALITY

Within the field of yogic scholarship, there are scholars who don't practise (Doniger 2013), scholars who do (Newcombe 2009), scholars whose own practice is key to their research and can be overly partisan (Langølen 2012), and scholars who are writing as much for a yogic audience as a scholarly one (Horton 2012). Each piece of research must justify its own terms of reference and ways of knowing. But as the academic field seeks to engage more openly with its researched audiences, there is an increasing tension between insider and outsider narratives that can be generative if researcher positionality is explicitly acknowledged and investigated.

The body is foundational to any form of yoga as a lived religious practice. Even the most esoteric of practices centres on the body: its placement, its ease, its breath, its relationship to its environment, and above all, the observation, control, cessation or appreciation of each practitioner's sensory world. And yet, even among such yoga scholars that address bodily experience directly, the most problematic and commonly unsubstantiated assumption is that both the body and the practice are universal points of reference. Unfortunately, most scholars are much more comfortable studying texts, and words, than moving bodies and their motivations. As Richard Carp writes:

Academic thought is produced by a specifically disciplined body, one that can tolerate sitting for hours in sterile rooms buzzing with the sound of fluorescent lights, listening to word after word after word of lecture after lecture.

(Carp 2001: 99)

Logically, then, most academic bodies are orthodox bodies, disciplined bodies, used to following rules and ignoring sensory needs, even if academic minds may be much more rebellious. Consistent with this reading, anecdotally, academic yoga practitioners tend to be followers of lineage.

Without some pre-existing knowledge of post-lineage yoga communities, I might never have been able to identify them as a productive site for research. Perhaps it is because of this, with some notable exceptions and ongoing investigations, that the story of post-lineage yoga is as yet largely untold. That story is about authenticity and religion as it is lived, rather than the ideals of community leaders and scriptural sources. It is part of what Robert Orsi calls 'the doctrines, rituals, or signs that men and women have picked up in their hands and are using to engage their immediate world' (Orsi 2003: 173).

While there are a number of such cultural markers that connect the people in this book, their defining characteristic is the practice of post-lineage yoga itself. From that data can be traced the intimate dependency of practice and ethics, identity and community, in the practices of emerging religious subcultures. As Graham Harvey writes, 'To do ritual is to be a member of a group. To be a member is to be shaped by the doing of ritual' (Harvey 2012: 110). The core ritual of post-lineage yoga is the practice itself.

The practice and its teaching are sensory, **kinetic** (pertaining to movement), relational and reflexive. I begin from the standpoint that mind and matter are inseparable and interdependent, co-creating each other (Sheets-Johnstone 2007: 297). In fact, not only is the body-mind inseparable, so is the thinking self and its environment: '**sensorimotor** simulations of external situations [involving both sensory and motor activity] are in fact widely implicated in human cognition' (Wilson 2002: 633). As such, my tendency is to focus on the fluid spaces of post-lineage practice, as sites of meaning-making in which internal and external, imagined and actual landscapes include the body of teacher, student, and lone practitioner, as intimate and interdependent stages for the evolution of each person's identity.

Yoga has been taught, as far as we can know, in a range of very different ways: in the one-to-one, even live-in intimacy of the *guru-śiṣya* relationship; in large, institutionalised ashrams; and more recently in secularised, consumer settings. There is a long history of textual manuals for specific audiences (Birch 2016), and diverse forms of media transmission have left their mark on the practice, from the development of photography to the rise of social media. But the most common way of learning yoga is still, in the modern era at least, through bodily, in person experiences, with the practice as demonstrated by teacher to student, and student to teacher. And yet, with few exceptions, very rarely has this vernacular process of teaching yoga to others been discussed in any systematic manner.

Given that the heart of this research concerns itself with group experiences, more relevant still is a strand of research into contagious aspects of human emotional expression. Nils Bubandt and Rane Willerslev (2015), as well as a wealth of work by Frans de Waal and collaborators (de Waal 2002, 2008; Preston and de Waal 2012), make a clear link between **mimesis** or mimicked movement, and empathy, cautioning that empathy itself can be a form of power over others. When we practise alone, what echoes, affordances and ghost gestures practise with us? And when we practise or teach others, what else is transmitted? Who are we as a result of practising together?

These questions are relevant not just for my participants, but also myself as researcher. My body is a presence in the data that must be accounted for. As Sheets-Johnstone says:

> movement offers us the possibility not only of formulating an epistemology true to the truths of experience, but of articulating a metaphysics true to the dynamic nature of the world and to the foundationally animated nature of life.
>
> (Sheets-Johnstone 2011: xix)

Within my analyses, I aim therefore to stay mindful of the meanings of these practices as they are experienced, and to document the internal, inter-human, inter-species and intra-ecological relationships of the practitioners themselves. Like Orsi and many others, I begin from the premise that there is much of value to be learned from the everyday rituals that people use to make meaning of their lives. After all, these everyday stories 'are forever at the edge of extinction, a reality that is effectively manipulated by the powerful' (Orsi 2013: 5).

My research position began in that which Graham Harvey describes as methodological guesthood: as a trusted guest who understood the most important community values and experiences, and could be relied upon to behave ethically and respectfully (Harvey 2014: 94). My position as a researcher evolved from guesthood, to service. As I will show, the practice of community service is one that holds practical, religious and political significance for post-lineage yoga. It is sometimes referred to as *karmayoga* (the yoga of action), or simply *sevā*, a word that has diverse and significant meanings across modern yoga subcultures (Beckerlegge 2015: 209). *Sevā* is considered to be equally, and at the same time, a practice of personal development and the freely offered currency that allows post-lineage events to thrive beyond commercial constraints.

I explored post-lineage events as an average participant would, not just eating, talking, resting and practising yoga with others, but serving the practical needs of this community in a number of capacities, by leading the occasional yoga session, helping in the kitchen and so on. This provided a much greater diversity of experiences, and facilitated a wider range of conversations with respondents. But including such acts of service that the community valued also enabled respondents to better understand my motives and reassure them that I was there to understand rather than expose them. And balancing my obligations to both the academic research process and the stories of my respondents was easier for myself to understand when I considered the ways in which I was serving both.

Just as considering my prior experience of diverse contemporary yoga *communities* was essential to developing my methodology, so my status as a prior participant in diverse yoga *practices* cannot be bracketed out, nor would it be productive to do so. Yoga, like any other physical discipline at any significant level of commitment is an incremental learnt process. This applies to the physical competence not just to achieve the various acts of movement, posture, breath and stillness, but also to the individualised knowledge of how to vary the practice according to one's embodied form, and the depth of awareness of sensations arising within the body. Long-term dedication to practice does not guarantee the most acrobatic results, but does confer a certain grace, ease, and skilful negotiation of its lived experience (Lussier-Ley 2010: 203).

My respondents struggled to convey how some aspects of another practitioner's experience are, for them, evident from observing their physical form in ways they are not for an observer without that embodied skillset. The same shape made by a body can be recognised by other practitioners as yoga or not depending on subtle contextual clues. And any number of other activities within the cultural ecology, from walking the site to chopping vegetables, could be understood as somehow 'yogic'. Put simply, practitioners both experience and observe yoga differently to non-practitioners.

My own long experience of various interoceptive and kinaesthetic practices confers a clear difference between my own, and many other academic bodies (McGuire 1990: 292). My own body, its flexibility, strength and sensitivity, is heavily implicated in the research process. I cannot pretend that it is neutral within the field. As Richard Carp writes:

> The anybody of the Academic body corresponds to the nowhere of Academic space. Yet the universality of academic knowledge is premised on the universality of the academic body.
>
> (Carp 2001: 99)

Beyond this research project there remains much more work to be done in examining the effect of what might be called a yoga body on the research of yoga in general. In my case, the body of the researcher is significantly implicated within the research. In that, it is no different from the body of the researcher in any experiential research (Giardina and Newman 2011: 526). My research data thus emerged as a unique iteration of the phenomena it describes, negotiated in the relationship of multiple bodily presences, the ecology surrounding those bodies, and all our practice histories (Giardina and Newman 2011: 530). My body alongside the bodies of my respondents, and our shared and separate history, habits and sensory fields, was a key site for my methodological experimentation.

CO-PRACTICE AS METHOD

My fieldwork activities were not otherwise unusual. Participant observation led to notes, photographs and onsite interviews, scans of event programmes and short snatches of video recording. Further interviews with event organisers were conducted after the events. My tiny camera and audio recorder could be pulled out at a moment's notice, and balanced almost anywhere. I wanted to know how the spaces of post-lineage yoga were shaped, how people moved through them and connected with each other. I was looking for common cultural reference points, common practices, common ways of teaching, and also, for what was considered to be normal, and what was innovative or taboo.

Fieldwork provided many examples of group practice, but I needed to get closer to the lived experience of individual practice, in a specific context and moment. As an experiment, I asked early respondents if they could begin a practice of yoga according to the emergent needs and practice of their day, and I would attempt to follow them, and then interview them about it.

Mimicking the respondent's practice gave me some insight into how my body responded to the practice, if not theirs. As mentioned earlier in this chapter, physical mimesis can be productive of an experience of high interpersonal attunement, enhancing the interview process. Simply stated, we sit like others and move like others when we want to attune to their way of being. In fieldwork, I had spent time moving and breathing with over forty different teachers and groups. Now, at the heart of the co-practice interviews, I quietly mimicked individual practices in intimate depth. Direct, face-to-face mirroring of the respondent felt too confronting, and rather than risk my presence dominating the data, I began to place myself instead just to one side and a little behind, copying rather than mirroring the respondent. A closer focus on the specific instance of practice was also enabled by playing back a recording of the practice during the subsequent interview. As the research evolved, unforeseeable challenges emerged when participants moved in ways that I could not follow, and each time I adapted the practice or abstained in a variety of ways. But in a very real sense, once established, the co-practice method was an immediate and ongoing source of surprisingly rich and dense data, as well as guaranteeing an immediate intimacy between researcher and researched that was evident to both.

Most importantly, this is not the naturally occurring data between multiple subjects that is common to much video analysis (Mondada 2012: 305), but a deliberate experiment in producing data with the researcher as participant. In all these ways, the bodily presence of both researcher and researched became assets in the data to be investigated, rather than problems to be solved (Wacquant 2014: 10).

Despite a partially shared practice repertoire and scope of aims, the circumstances of the co-practice process were unique. Yoga teachers are often mimicked by yoga students in the normal process of knowledge transmission to the group, but this is at least ostensibly in the service of the evolving student and culture. Yoga practitioners, especially teachers, might share less formal co-practice sessions on occasion, blending individual need into shared aims and a group practice. But the experience of having one's individual practice shadowed by another practitioner is *extremely* unusual. Most respondents referred in some way to the unexpected and powerful sense of intimacy it provoked. Paraphrasing my respondent **Sivani Mata** (Case study 4): her usual practice involves her in relationship with her altar, and the relationship as a whole held within a wider circle of benevolent protection. In sharing her morning ***pūjā*** (ritual practice) with me, there was an additional presence in the form of myself as interviewer. This formed a shadow gaze to her own, multiplied by the gaze of my camera. There was, as a result, a field containing the respondent and the altar in intimate relationship, witnessed by the gaze of the researcher. This multiple gaze was itself held by the gaze of the camera. For my respondent, this was also all held within the circle of divine protection or presence. The result for her was an off-centring, a feeling of being pulled slightly out of one's usual orbit, and an unprecedented level of intimacy and being witnessed.

None of my respondents experienced the intimacy of the co-practice event negatively, but I became aware of needing to respond ethically and honourably to the emotional intimacy as it emerged. There is some precedent for this way of working outside of the academy. A very effective but resource-intense therapeutic technique called Intensive Interaction, as introduced by Jefferies (2009) and reviewed by Hutchinson and Bodicoat (2015), uses physical mimesis to encourage non-verbal autistic people into social interaction, communication, and deeper relationship with care staff and families. Although the theory and practice of Intensive Interaction was, at best, tangential to the research, I became aware that my familiarity with it also informed the co-practice lens of the research.

More widely, the issues of yoga in transmission are reflected in the method. Just as the choice of media generates certain forms of practice data, so media choice privileges certain aspects of cultural transmission. And the presence of bodies with histories, abilities and tendencies, as well as who leads movement and who follows, is a vector for interpersonal power dynamics within the transmission of yoga, just as it is generative of power dynamics within the research relationship.

NOTATION

Because of the diversity of practices, schools, sources and lineages involved in post-lineage yoga, there is no standard notation or typology of yogic ***mudrā*** (hand gesture) or *āsana*, by name, description or graphic.

After developing the co-practice method, the most challenging aspect of my research was deciding how to notate the kinetic and interoceptive, performative and lived practice to enable its comparison. It became clear in the fieldwork that the diversity of post-lineage practice is reflective of a similar diversity of aims and experiences. Beyond the visual data, interoceptive data is by its nature highly subjective, and its analysis relies on developing a richness of vocabulary and thickness of sense impressions in what Eduardo Viveiros de Castro has called a 'good enough description' that retains its natural paradoxes (2014: 15).

Standard dance notation is usually derived from the work of Rudolph Laban or that of Joan and Rudolf Benesh. Laban's Eukinetics is:

> the study of rhythm, phrasing and dynamics in dance. It categorises four basic factors in motion: Weight: Light or Strong; Time: Sustained or Sudden; Flow: Free or Bound; Space: Flexible or Direct.
>
> (Athreya 2001)

Benesh notation, and its simplified version, Motif, are constructed like a musical score, as we can see in Royal Academy of Dance (2014) and Guest (2007) respectively.

But yoga is not dance, and in order to faithfully notate kinetic practice and include such vital elements as breath flow and internal alignment, a range of systems, including practitioners' own individualised notation practices, contributed to my recording of the practice. My notation reflects all those aspects of the practice that I wished to analyse: the shapes, movements and pacing of practice; interoceptive aims and experience; orientation to the ecology of practice; and the processes of transmission.

Beyond an initial recording of data, my notation system became of vital use in representing examples of practice in my writing. It further became clear that a notation system designed to capture and represent not just the movements, but the intentions and other qualities of post-lineage practice, is applicable to many other similar datasets. When I shared my notes with a few other scholars, we realised that it was adaptable to many such movement practices, and could enable innovative methods of comparison between them.

A similar system produced within the study of a community with a narrower range of common practice would still be a significant innovation in the field of yoga studies. But it is the very diversity of post-lineage practice data that necessitated such an adaptable, modifiable notation system to

Notation key

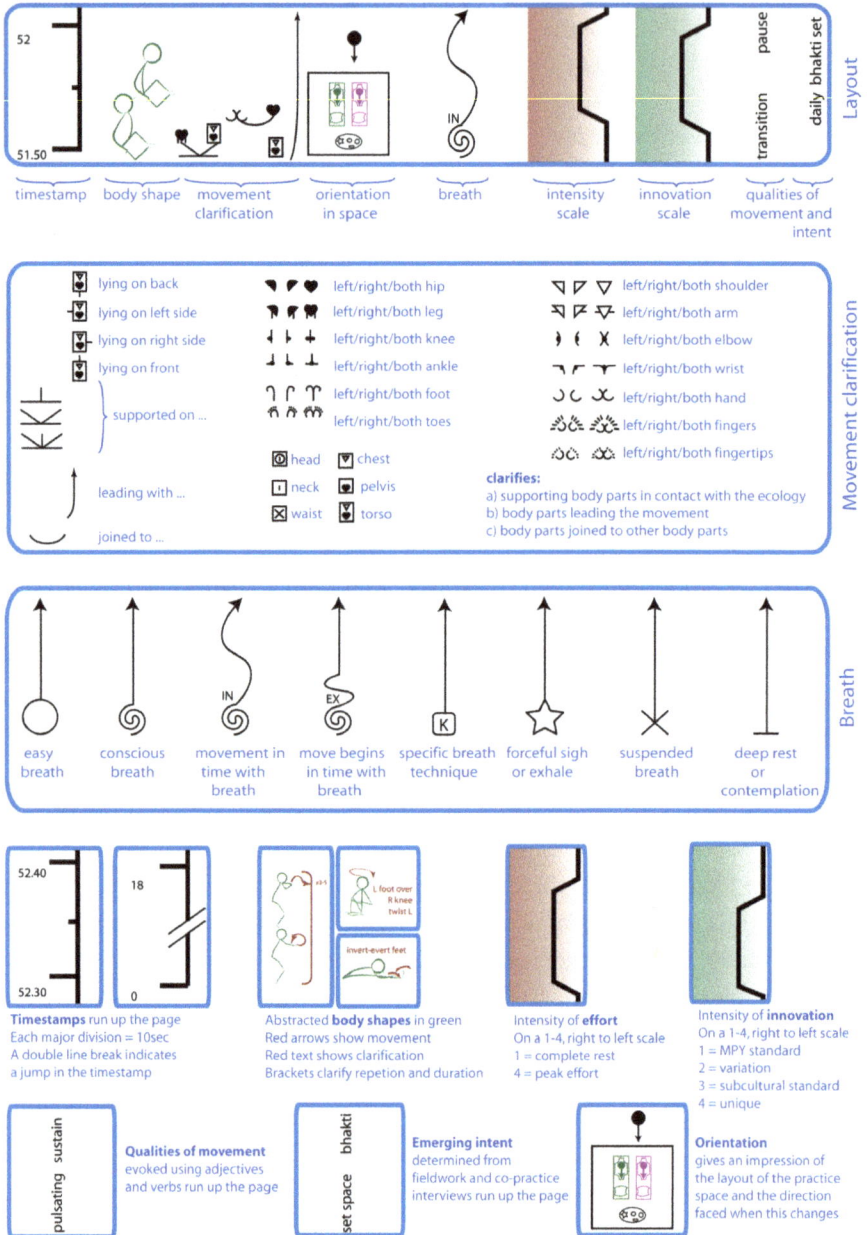

Figure 2.1
Notation key

emerge. Thus I include here a clear explanation of motivations and major features that the reader can use to navigate the notation used in the rest of the book, and in the confidence that it will be of further use to future research.

Reading each line of the notation in Figure 2.1 from left to right, the first element is a simple timestamp, followed by an abstract visual representation of the shape held by the respondent's body (in green) in that moment. The various colours are included only to make the diagrams more readable. During the case studies, the camera ran constantly, and thus the timestamp there corresponds closely to the length of the practice. During fieldwork however, I filmed only short fragments of sessions and other scenes of interest, so some of the examples in this book have no timestamp at all. The notation system is designed to be modular, so that a researcher can add or drop elements, as is most appropriate for the data at hand.

(Red) arrows indicate directions of movement, brackets indicate a repeated movement, and occasional text is added for clarification of, for example, which foot is represented. Any verbal asides or external noises are also represented here. This line of the notation lacks the exact precision of Benesh or Laban, but can be read much more easily by a non-expert. It allows for a more immediate impression of the overall arc of the bodily shape held by the respondent in each moment.

The following example is from **Tanya**'s practice (Case study 5). We can see that the timestamp runs from 11 minutes 20 seconds to 11 minutes 30, and then compresses the next three minutes, jumping to 14 minutes 20. In Figure 2.2 we can see Tanya is kneeling, leaning forward to her timer and

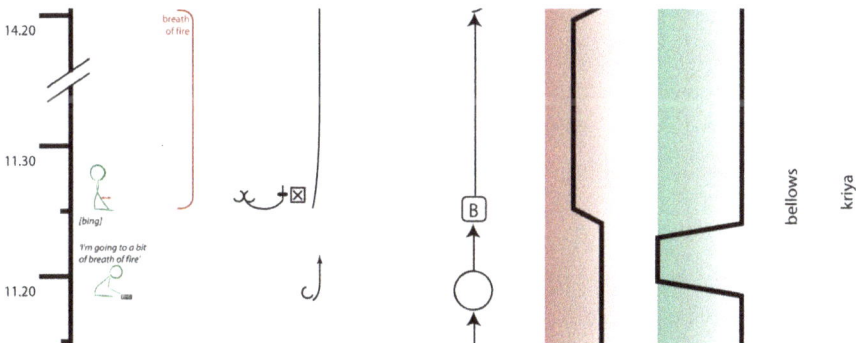

Figure 2.2
Case Study 5: Breath of Fire

saying a few words. The sound of the timer is represented with a 'bing', and for the rest of the time shown, Tanya is sitting on her feet, hands on her knees, with her abdomen moving in and out in the repeated practice called 'breath of fire'.

The next line clarifies three aspects of the movement and posture that emerged as most useful to analysis. These are: which body parts are in contact with the ground (suggesting their relationship to ecology); which body part(s) are leading (suggesting somatic focus); and whether any body parts are in contact with each other (suggesting intrapersonal connection). This part of the notation is most influenced by Motif notation. However, the Motif symbols, while fast to sketch, are difficult as a non-specialist to tell apart, relying on counting multiple hash lines on a stave. For this system it was worth creating more distinctive shapes for my own ease and that of the reader, using the key above. This line allows for more detail to be shown of these three specific aspects. In the above example, the line shows that Tanya does not change her position with regard to contact with the ground, but she does bring her hands to her knees. When changing the timer, she leads with her right hand, and during the breath of fire, her abdomen is leading all movement.

The next line represents the respondent's orientation to the space. At the start of notation, this contains a simplified representation of the physical environment, which is repeated only each time the respondent changes position relative to the overall space. For this reason, individual notation extracts in this book may not include it. When it is relevant, it also shows the researcher's position within the practice space. Elsewhere on the line, arrows are used to denote a change in orientation by the respondent without a change in position relative to space. This line allows for an impression of the practice space overall, and the respondent's movement relative to ecology. In Figure 2.3, from Sivani Mata's practice (Case study 4), we can see her moving from sitting to hands and knees. At first, she turns away from me, and we can see her voiced discomfort with that position. Eventually, she reorients herself entirely in the space, which we can see from the inclusion of a diagram of the space. This also shows us the space is crowded with furniture and ritual paraphernalia.

The next line is the most unique in notation, as dance rhythms are almost always oriented to a musical tempo, while in yoga, movement and stillness alike are most frequently oriented to the tempo of the respondent's breath. In this line, breath notation describes three interdependent factors. Initial symbols denote the respondent's breath pattern, such as a

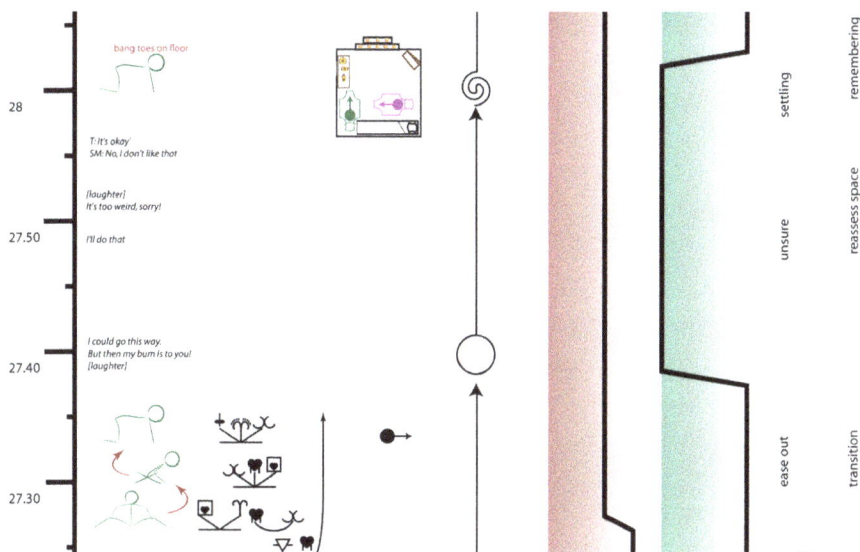

Figure 2.3
Case study 4: Negotiating space

circle for easy, normal breathing, spiral for conscious, deliberate breathing, or a horizontal line for a suspended breath. An arrow leading from that symbol extends for the length of time that pattern is held. The vertical bar of that arrow has a horizontal wave if the movement and breath are in time. That wave returns to a straight vertical if the movement begins on the breath, but does not continue to hold that pace. Finally, a small 'IN' or 'EX' is added if the movement always begins on an inhale or exhale. This line allows notation of a foundational element of contemporary yoga practice. The many different ways breath and movement are combined can here be represented. In the above example, the breath of Sivani Mata (Case study 4), shifts from a non-deliberate to a deliberate pattern as she settles into a new position.

The next two lines of notation are scales. They are impressionistic, referring to my own, informed understanding of interoceptive and relational aspects of the practice, respectively. The first suggests the relative intensity in intent and movement at a given moment compared to that specific practice overall, as I both experienced it and as understood from the post-practice interviews. Thus, lying down resting would rate a '1', and a complex arm balance necessitating intense concentration would rate a '4'. Some practices describe a series of waves, some sustain a higher level of intensity overall. This line confers a sense of the overall intensity pattern of mental and physical effort, what we might call the cost of the practice, but it is approximate, and subjective, and does not lend itself to such nuances as practices of intense concentration that are conducted in a simple seated position, which rated a '2', for example.

The second line suggests the relative innovation of a given element of practice compared to the subculture as a whole. This scale is dependent on prior knowledge, obtained during my fieldwork, of how far each practice element diverges from the norms of the modern postural yoga mainstream, from the most dominant lineages, and from the subculture as a whole. Some elements are familiar from the most common modern postural yoga standards, in accepted or variant forms. These rate as a '1' and '2' here respectively. Some elements are unusual within the wider yoga cultural repertoire, but are often practised within the research subculture. These rate as a '3'. Some are unique to the respondent's practice or teaching. These rate as a '4'. In practice, the boundaries between categories of innovation are porous, and again, this is a numerical scale that describes a subjective impression. This line thus confers a sense of the overall pattern of orthodoxy and innovation, what we might consider as evidence of cultural evolution within the practice. Either line could be replaced by another useful metric, but within this project, my informed impressions of the intensity and innovation were the most useful to record. In Figure 2.4, Uma (Case study 3), pauses to rearrange her clothing, before effort resumes, in a series of spinal movements that shift between variations on a form of *uḍḍīyana bandha* (abdominal 'lock') and wriggling movements that are all her own.

The final two lines of notation are entirely qualitative. They consist of a series of descriptive words. The first evokes an observation of the quality of the movement, using terms such as pulsating, sustained or precise. The second recalls cues from context both internal and external to the practice to suggest the intent of each element.

This part of the notation was conducted with detailed reference to the co-practice interviews, and fieldwork notes of group practices taught by the respondent. Taken together, the lines enable both a thickening of sense description, and a first analysis of the relationship between practice and intent. Either line could be replaced by a different descriptive field if more appropriate to a different research project. In the above example, movements with a pumping and lubricating quality are used with the intention of raising energy and heat in the body.

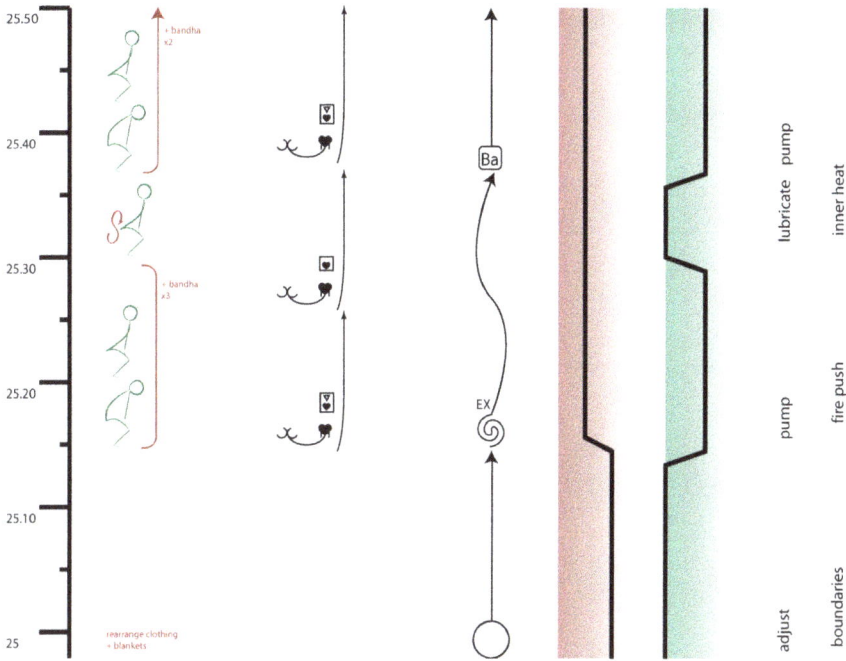

Figure 2.4
Case study 3: Uḍḍīyana bandha

Each element of the notation facilitated further analysis. Practices can be printed to be visualised as a whole, enabling consideration of them as distinct case studies. Differences between practices, and therefore case studies, are also immediately apparent when visually comparing their notation. The notation performs a coding function, as common elements or themes are easy to find both within and between practices. At the same time the coherence of each practice as a distinct, holistic part of the data is maintained. Most existing dance notation systems dedicate the most space to lines for each body part, rendering movement in space with more precision. In contrast, this notation system is more concerned with the line of the body in space as a whole, and dedicates space to lines for the many essential factors of practice that do not concern shape, such as breath, intensity, innovation and intent, thus enabling their synchronous comparison. As a result, as we will see, I was able to much more accurately relate movement and intention to interoceptive and somatic experience.

SOME FAULT LINES AND CONCLUSIONS

Within the process of analysis, it became clear that as the different lenses of text, fieldwork and co-practice interviews were brought to bear on the research, the data produced was not uniform. Processes of **interoception** (awareness of one's internal physiological condition), performance and transmission did not map neatly on to each other. To use a musical analogy, a score that represented the movements of a given yoga session would be on a different line of a score from one representing its transmitted understanding, or its interoceptive experience. As my notation shows, different lines are synchronous and can be compared, but are not coterminous. Different methodological tools were not merely lenses considering the same subject, they were examining overlapping but distinct forms of subject matter. The lacunae formed from the partial correspondence of movement to experience, and movement to transmitted experience, are key to understanding the incremental and individualised ways in which movement cultures both reproduce themselves and allow for those errors or echoes in reproduction that produce innovation and diversity (Holloway 2003: 1971). In the gap between the bodies of teacher and student, method, aim and experience, transformation can occur. In the fault lines between the bodies of researcher and respondent, participant and target of observation, lie everyday fieldwork experiences such as fatigue, confusion, and misunderstanding, but also a deeper understanding of the crevasses of possible neurological and physical difference that the transmission structures of interoceptive and kinetic practice aim to overcome.

The research design was necessarily and deliberately productive of the partial truths and experimental conclusions familiar to qualitative research as a whole. The research was designed to provoke as many questions as answers and to explore and test new theories for the study of lived and moved religious practice, a field as yet in early development. The question of how to more clearly analyse intra- and interpersonal transmission of physical practice is not fully answered by this research project, and as such survives the research process to become part of its conclusion.

My methodology is more than experimental. Its primary method is the experiment, in the form of a comparative analysis of its diverse methodological lenses, which continually refers back to its data target in the search for increased clarity in answering the research question. As such, it is 'real world research' (Robson 2002) in action, as productive of new methodology as it is of new data.

3
Coming together

While post-lineage is a widespread phenomenon, this research centres on a specific and shifting network of post-lineage, non-commercial yoga devotees who gather at a series of annual events. By mapping levels of engagement, roles and interpersonal relationships in this post-lineage subculture, we bring into focus a community that is ever in flux, and includes post-lineage beginners, committed teacher-practitioners, organisers and activists.

Above all, the communal rituals of post-lineage yoga are fuelled and inspired by the dedicated, long term practice of many of its key members: the yoga teachers, crew and musicians who gather each summer to share, work and as some put it, 'feed their souls' in order to better serve their own local communities. In this book I focus on three events: Colourfest, Santosa and Sundara; and six case studies of key actors in this subcultural network. Those individuals – **Veronika**, **Christopher**, Uma, Sivani Mata, Tanya and **Nicole** – are the focus of Part II. Uma is also included as the founder and organiser of Santosa, and Tanya, and her husband, John, are included as the founders and organisers of Sundara. All of them are dedicated practitioners and gifted teachers, but their inclusion as case studies does not reflect any hierarchy of approval over any other teacher or practitioner. Just as I chose Colourfest, Santosa and Sundara as an interesting cluster of highly coherent and interdependent events, I chose those case studies that were the most interesting, thought-provoking, and highly relevant to understanding the community, its history and its practice.

During the research, I met others who were Sanskrit scholars, independent researchers, activists and philosophers. All these people were highly educated, widely read, or simply profoundly experienced in decades of practice. Some of them are quoted herein, but for simplicity, only a few are introduced by name and history. As founders and organisers of Colourfest, both **Rowan** and **Robbie**, for example, have their own complex stories and depths of applicable knowledge. Apart from Rowan and Robbie, I interviewed **Ian**, who is quoted later, because his One Spirit Ashram Kitchen is a fascinating development that connects this community to much bigger activist networks. Although he does practise and teach an interesting synthesis of Ashtanga, Hatha and **Kundalini Yoga**,[1] he does so much more occasionally, focusing recently on his ministry for the One Spirit Interfaith ministry network.

Also mentioned by name is **Trishula**, the founder and organiser of her own event, the Beltane Bhakti Gathering. She is a key figure within the community, and her husband is a well-known ***bhakti*** (devotional) musician and producer. Together they model and promote inter-lineage collaboration and the importance of both social justice and service. Understanding Trishula's role is instrumental in understanding both the specificity of this subculture, and the wider processes of post-lineage collaboration. Yet her individual practice focuses almost exclusively on *bhakti*, and my case studies are confined to those practitioners with a more eclectic practice.

In this network, long-term practitioners are always in the majority, but they necessarily come into contact with those having rather different aims and experiences. Interpersonal relationships sustain a post-lineage subculture's overall coherence. Changing roles and levels of engagement help determine its rate of evolution. Before we turn to the detail of specific events, and specific case studies, it is useful to describe some of the typical journeys to and through post-lineage yoga.

COMING TO POST-LINEAGE YOGA FOR THE FIRST TIME

It is important to remember that although this is a participative subculture, these events are also targeted at a population of less engaged members, who attend the events, partake of their offerings, and to an extent, contribute the largest financial support (Jenkins and Carpentier 2013: 271). Thus, organisers must balance offerings that will benefit the community, with offerings that have wider appeal.

In one session of Japa Yoga (chanting practice) at Colourfest, the teacher mentions how pop versions of the Gāyatrī Mantra, such as the one by Deva

---

1 Yoga practices inspired by and developed from the teachings of Yogi Bhajan, focused on esoteric development and raising Kuṇḍalinī.

Premal that inspired at least one television soundtrack (Glendening 2012), lack the 'power' of more traditional versions but serve to 'draw people in' to a deeper consideration of the possibilities of chanting as a practice. The view that there are levels of engagement with yoga that one moves through, charmed by more accessible offerings into a more profound involvement, is extremely commonly held here. It may not reflect the typical experiences of a majority of casual yoga practitioners. But it resonates with the audience attending such events precisely because it describes their own ongoing journeys to what they consider to be more profound, more authentic, and more diverse yoga practices.

This is a journey that these events are designed in many ways to enable. Its hopeful pragmatism complicates any easy separation between commercial and non-commercial methods of transmission in contemporary yoga. Indeed, it is a great mistake to assume that any teacher's knowledge of yoga practice is only as extensive as their teaching output. In the conversations happening in post-lineage communities, yoga teachers commonly discuss the problem of how to engage the most casual of practitioners in a wider diversity of offerings beyond the culturally accessible format of *sūrya namaskāra,* stretching, breathing and relaxation.

Significant numbers of people attend the events profiled here as part of a first introduction to post-lineage yoga. The vast majority of these are, however, *already yoga teachers,* looking for something not found in their experiences of mainstream yoga so far. Most commonly they seek support for dealing with more negative experiences in other yoga spaces, or seek resources to further develop their personal and teaching practice. The structure of many yoga teacher trainings involves little post-graduation support, and the large number of graduates and an often competitive market can leave teachers feeling very isolated (Goldberg 2015; Hargreaves 2018). For first-time attendees of this kind, the most predictable rewards of these events are increased solidarity, new friendships and some refreshing of their practice repertoires. For many, this is enough, but for others, as described in the next section, this transforms over time into a deeper affinity and commitment to the community.

The place of these events within a wider network of camps and small festivals in Britain also attracts a few people whose previous engagement with yoga is minimal. Their affinity is more to the festival subculture than to yoga. Post-lineage yoga in those cases is an experiment in experience among many others. Without an established, self-reflexive practice of some kind however, the group sessions on offer here are more confusing to navigate. Making a choice between subcultural activities is more difficult when an attendee does not share the subcultural reference points of, for example, 'masculine' versus 'feminine' forms of movement, or the object and intent of *bhakti* activities, and there is always the risk of not knowing one's body well enough to make the individually appropriate decisions that avoid physical strain.

Post-lineage yoga, its adherents agree, is a product of regular individual practice, and a significant level of reflexivity. This level of commitment is of a different order than that of the casual practitioner who might attend a yoga class once a week, and of a different kind than the devoted practitioner aiming to faithfully reproduce modern postural yoga at home. The intuition involved in finding a personalised practice appropriate to the evolving nature of one's lived experience, day after day, year after year, is vital for the committed post-lineage practitioner.

Almost all yoga students first learn a practice by rote before ever learning how to choose between practice elements. In post-lineage practice these elements prescribed by external authority are ideally, as I have explained, confirmed with the authority of the inner self, and are tested against group norms. But while the beginner to *yoga* might be acquiring new habits of movement, the transition from modern postural to *post-lineage* yoga is as likely to involve breaking existing movement habits as forming new ones.

All of the established post-lineage practitioners I spoke to had begun their journey into the practice by in some way moving beyond more authoritarian yoga schools. Despite this all of the case studies profiled later in this book have repertoires that include at least as many movements learned by rote through lineage as those intuited and shared through peer networks. Over the page, for example, are very similar *vinyāsa* variations from Ashtanga Yoga in Veronika, Christopher and Tanya's practice repertoires, in Case Studies 1, 2 and 5 (Figures 7 and 8).

One of the most common initial drives behind a significant commitment to post-lineage yoga, is reflecting on some form of adverse experience with modern postural yoga. As I explained in Chapter 1, this is often complicated by the other adverse life experiences that the practitioner seeks to manage or heal through individual practice: the ongoing effects of everything from childhood trauma to torn ligaments; from prostrate problems to bereavement. Such practitioners attempt to remake the self through a crucible of experience that distils personal and spiritual rewards from any experience (Robertson and Wildcroft 2017: 98).

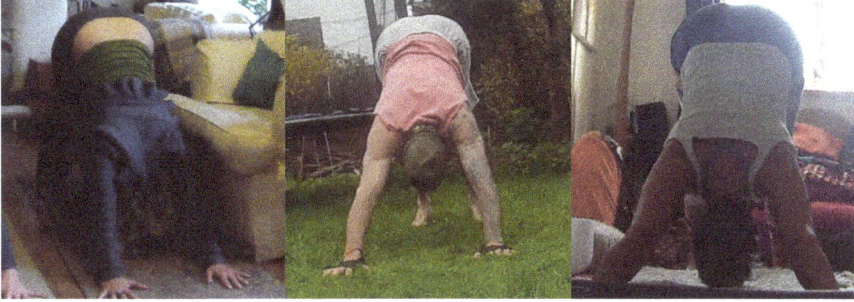

Figure 3.1
Case studies 1, 2 and 5: Vinyāsa variations

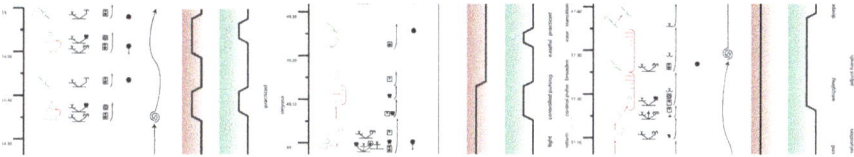

Figure 3.2
Case studies 1, 2 and 5: Vinyāsa variations

Thus, although today the subculture under consideration also includes members who maintain allegiances to one of the more open yoga lineages, engaging in what we might call a kind of intra-yoga interfaith, at the heart of post-lineage impetus to practice, is a transformation of diverse and often mundane forms of adverse experience. And this holds true for many of those more casual attendees of these events, who will also often be attracted to post-lineage practice in the hope of healing something in their own histories. It is for this reason that re-mapping the body is a common intention to practice, un-training postural habits as often as training them.

From its inception, modern postural yoga has sought to improve bodies, and developed methods of conditioning to train bodies for that improvement (Alter 2006: 760). In this, it is part of a much wider, and long-established trans-cultural trend (Gilman 2014: 69; Jesson 2017). But in the process of learning to re-map the body and its history of practice, the locus of authority, and thus the location of the authentic voice of the self, can be difficult to navigate (Ulland 2012: 86). The cultural stories imparted with practice have complex roots and carry currents of interpersonal and socio-political power.

The scholar Elizabeth Behnke (1997: 187–8) extends the work of Husserl to explore the idea of 'ghost gestures': sedimented and internalised qualities that structure our potential future movement landscape. Movement educators often describe the missing movement ranges that each individual loses over time as a kind of sensorimotor amnesia. Seen in this light, inherited cultural habits of movement involve blind spots equivalent to a kind of sensorimotor cognitive dissonance. This is as true of someone whose spine adjusts to support the now absent weight of a bag carried on the same shoulder for years, as it is true of someone whose body has adapted to anticipate the daily pre-dawn performance of *sūrya namaskāra* characteristic of the Ashtanga Vinyasa Yoga system.

While a particular practitioner may decide that any such habits have become life-enhancing or life-constraining, the first task is recognising they exist. And while modern postural yoga includes various observational techniques for recognising habits formed in everyday life, individual lineages evolve fewer techniques for recognising any negative aspects to habits formed *within the practices they prescribe.* The very point of modern postural yoga is to imprint the student body indelibly with a particular set of habits that the teaching hierarchy has found to be beneficial.

As I will show, dedicated post-lineage yoga practitioners have developed the self-awareness to resist at least some of the dominant dynamics of modern postural yoga, but the resulting dance of effort and ease, resilience training and self-nourishment inherent to the practice is a delicate one for beginners to navigate. Nonetheless, these events are an opportunity for many to engage in activities outside one's comfort zone, leading to new experiences of self, and relationship, and new ways of moving through the world by experiencing temporary **entrainment**[2] with others with very different lifestyles. As Uma says of Santosa:

> Maybe they're just getting tasters. But the tastes they're getting! [LC] is one of the best Sanskrit teachers in the whole country. That is her thing. And she's sitting there in a tent sharing it with people who've never done it before.

As a result, among the curious and casual attendees, there continue to be new people willing to make a commitment to increasing reflexivity in

---

2 Often unconscious synchronisation of organic movement such as gesture and heart rate to an external rhythm.

practice, and increasing engagement with the post-lineage community as a source of both solidarity, and new practice resources.

MAKING THE JOURNEY TO COMMITTED TEACHER-PRACTITIONER

As I explained in Chapter 1, not only are the majority of attendees at these post-lineage events already yoga teachers, a high proportion of attendees contribute teaching or other forms of service at each event itself. At Santosa it is estimated that for every attendee who is not teaching on site, there is another who is, plus another on an 'elf' ticket, contributing at least 4 hours of practical service a day. At many events, the casual attendee is outnumbered as much as two to one by committed members of the community. Only at Colourfest is the proportion of working community members significantly smaller than that of paying, often less invested participants.

As a person's level of engagement in the post-lineage community increases, they start to take on more vital service roles for the events. They become trusted figures, and are more likely to be asked or allowed to teach. Each organiser controls which teachers, musicians and other facilitators are given space on the schedule. Organisers differ in their criteria, but at every event included in my research, the quality of one's professional offering was not the only factor. A willingness to perform the most mundane of *sevā*, and a commitment to inclusive teaching, and to warm relationships with the rest of the community, are essential. A few highly respected, well-known teachers will be invited to teach at the events before ever attending, and even compensated for doing so. But the majority of teachers here pass through the same informal tests, proving their commitment to the ethical standards and community cohesion of the network before they come into a position to teach on a regular basis, and thus influence the shared repertoire of yoga practice.

Some yoga teachers fail that test:

> They show up and it's muddy, and they can't look very glamorous, and they've got to shit in a composting toilet and eat rice and dal. [...] They're welcome to come, but they tend not to be very successful in the teaching.
>
> (Uma)

For those who do become established members of this subculture, post-lineage yoga events provide them with some modest economic advantages, in accessing a wider pool of potential students to fill their own retreats and courses. But all established community members consider such rewards to be a minor consideration. They talk frequently of 'filling themselves up' for the year (Santosa 2014). Reconnecting in this way with the *saṃgha* or practice community also reinforces their dedication to experimentation and reflexivity.

For this majority group, both the shared subculture and individual practice also function as a refuge and wellspring of resistance to a wider culture that many still experience as more or less hostile:

> You go out into the world and sometimes things can really feel like a physical blow. [...] And so in a sense, you're cleansing your body of those physical blows by trying to get back to that original source.
>
> (Veronika, Case study 1)

> Capitalism is the sort of – almost the arch anti-yogic event. It's separatist, nihilistic materialism of the worst kind.
>
> (Christopher, Case study 2)

The mundane world, like the mundane self, is never wholly escapable (Orsi 2012: 153). But many practitioners here seek not just symptom management and simple wellbeing, but a reclamation of agency, active resistance to high social levels of anxiety (PlanC 2015), and a transformation of the idea of universal healing into cyclical rhythms of self-maintenance.

> I dislocated my ankle a few weeks ago anyway. And I've got a broken toe on the other foot from a couple of years back, so I've always got to do some hip maintenance stuff.
>
> (Veronika, Case study 1)

For such members of the subculture, the support of a post-lineage *saṃgha* or learning community is vital to their ongoing ability to thrive and teach within a wider socio-political system that routinely under-resources those – mostly women – in self-employed creative and caring professions such as teaching yoga. A deeper connection to this post-lineage subculture is often provoked by negative experiences in life or in yoga. It is always accompanied by a significant commitment to self-reflexive practice. It is also consistent with a certain alienation with mainstream societal norms.

One common desire among female teachers of post-lineage yoga is for a less-patriarchal form of yoga than that which they first encountered

(Westoby 2018; Cixous and Sellers 1994: 62), even to heal from abusive encounters with male yoga teachers (Lucas 2016). As Uma says in Case study 3: 'we're all good daughters of patriarchy, so we're used to doing what we're told'.

For Uma and many others, a practice more overtly attuned to the experiences and histories of women can heal a wounded female self, broken female body and corrupted world-as-goddess in one. Post-lineage yoga practice for these practitioners attempts to reclaim a supposed unpredictable wild self from the more normative female self of mainstream culture (Cixous 1976: 876). But in doing so, they are inevitably wresting self-nourishment from bodily practices created through patriarchal discipline (Ginot 2010: 23), further marked by the historical struggle between a subaltern Indian and an oppressive British culture.

> My practice would be three hours. And over an hour of that would be *āsana*. [...] I became anaemic and then I just did **yoganidrā** [guided relaxation] for over a year.
>
> (Sivani Mata, Case study 4)

As a result, in post-lineage yoga, the narratives surrounding this transformation often speak of imperfect solutions, of managing or reconciling rather than healing, and of carrying what cannot be fixed (Devine 2015). In post-lineage yoga, the practice is a space in which to reframe as much as transform the self and its world.

The making of shared subcultural experiences here is laminar: a mundane chronic pain or a deeper root of suffering is laminated in layers of experiences of ease and reconciliation, each one intimately formed not just from movement and stillness, but from the time and place of practice, and its narrative framing and instruction. The newly transformed identity of the teacher-practitioner, and the reframed meaning of their experiences are formed through accretion, hardened through a process of witnessing and storying the self. When these newly coherent selves and transformed experiences are repeated for others, deeply individualised experiences can be fitted into a wider cultural repertoire of stories. Publicly performed identities extrude from privately emergent identities, formed in individual practice, and translated into the language of common subcultural association. Deeply felt stories emerge from re-enchanted spaces, carried by deeply practised bodies, with the power to change others.

The most visible reward of long-term, individual post-lineage yoga practice, or indeed any committed movement practice, is a unified and coherent quality of presence and movement. Established members of the subculture are often recognisable by the way they move even outside of the practice. At Colourfest, waiting for a dance session to begin, one teacher pointed out to me that among over a thousand attendees, experienced practitioners could be recognised by how they walked across the site towards the practice space, even before their faces came into focus.

Self-reflexive practices combine over time to form embodied repertoires of physical grace. Overall movement becomes more efficient and intuitive, but also diverse and expressive. In the everyday rhythms of individual practice, such transformation comes from repetition. After one movement, the practitioner is a person who has carried out the movement. After many repetitions, the practitioner is a person who is partly defined by doing the movement: a person who practises yoga, rather than a person who has practised it. Eventually authority over that movement is also conferred: the practitioner becomes the author of this variation of the movement. But the practice continues to evolve.

This deeply introspective, fluid experience is what drives committed, long-term practice, even if the initial impulse to explore the subculture is very different. It explains the connections post-lineage yoga teachers make between the personal, the communal, the political and the ecological. At the heart of post-lineage yoga, as a practice that combines devotion, self-awareness and discipline, is a need to remake oneself within the world: to reconfigure our most fundamental relations within a more than human web. As Uma is fond of quoting: 'You may dissolve in contemplation, as salt does in water, but there's something more that must happen' (Ded and Hoskote 2013: 30).

THE TENSION BETWEEN CHARISMA AND PRAGMATISM FOR THE ORGANISER AND ACTIVIST

Within the tangled web of relationships supporting this post-lineage subculture, smaller networks can be differentiated in line with these same levels of engagement. The wider pool of casual attendees is the most weakly connected within the subculture, the most dependent on the core community at its heart for access to subcultural events, and also the most connected to the cultural mainstream. Entangled and somewhat inseparable from it is the inner network of dedicated and reflexive yoga teachers as detailed in the previous section. These yoga teachers are also supported by and overlap with other established community members, including site crew and *bhakti* musicians, who may also have their own individual practice, less visible within the repertoires of shared spaces.

Deeper still is the much tinier network of event organisers. Their roles involve a further level of investment in the subculture, and a different kind of reward and risk. Organisers are among the most invested, not only in the subculture, but in the most highly reflexive of individual practices. In post-lineage yoga, as in most informal networks, local individuals such as these function as gatekeepers to community events and thus cultural resources (Castells 2011: 773). Despite the informal, interpersonal nature of affiliation here, this is not an insular subculture. It maintains more direct links to India in particular than are prevalent in North American yoga subcultures, as exemplified by Brown (2015). A number of teachers make yearly trips to India, and a few are Indian by birth. Trishula, who organises the Beltane Bhakti Gathering, also performs at other events with the Babaji Temple Singers, and is the daughter of a Brahmin family. A small but significant number of other teachers are British Hindus. These teachers have diverse histories, dependent on the complex intersectionality of their socio-political status.

Trishula has fond memories of childhood Durga *pūjās* in Sheffield, accompanied by acute recollections of being forbidden by her gender to perform certain ritual acts. She speaks movingly of her debut as a public ritualist, enabled by white, male priests of the Babaji lineage. She says:

> When I offered the water, as I was doing that, I really felt my dad so strong because I had been so many times standing in the crowd when he has done that. And so there was a moment of how our own relationship with our parents is so mixed.

As a result, she is very aware of how gatekeepers structure access to religious knowledge.

Contemporary yoga appears to be dominated by the many commercial and standardised, large scale interpretations of yoga which monetise subcultural and traditional cultural resources through mechanisms marked by exoticisation, exploitation and superficial engagement (Oh and Sarkisian 2012: 301; Carrette and King 2013: 117). In contrast, gatekeepers in this post-lineage network at least are characterised by their length of dedication to the practice and lack of interest in financial wealth. But prejudices of many kinds can be born in any situation where people are free to choose the intuitive comfort of consorting with people they already admire or resemble (Caldarelli and Catanzaro 2012: 75–6).

While all organisers expressed enthusiasm for their role, the personal cost of running events is also high. Every year more than one considers taking a 'fallow year' to recover, but almost always finds the inspiration to continue anyway, during the dreaming and planning of the winter season. Those organisers who were open with me about their financial invest-ment in their events confirmed that they pay themselves far more rarely than others, despite spending most of the year planning and preparing for a single event. As Rowan says of Colourfest:

> We're spending money on those things because we want the event to be immense. But [...] we've put the equivalent of five years of our lives into the festival and it's not helping us do what we need in our life. It's not helping us to put our kids through school.

Added to this, organisers seem more likely to encounter a level of inter-personal conflict that leads in some cases to them leaving core teams and creating new events. For the subculture as a whole, this is positive, as it leads to events multiplying, increasing choice. But in private, some at the heart of the subculture expressed enduring regret at the loss of friend-ship or personal investment involved. Falling out and moving on can have a greater impact on organisers. While they are among the most visible and connected figures in the community network, organisers can experi-ence a form of localised micro-celebrity, in which their self-presentation is bound to the feel of the event as a whole, rendering their experiences on site subordinate to their own image.

Post-lineage yoga avoids the institutionalisation of charisma that is characteristic of lineages and brands. But its overlapping affinity groups and communities of practice are still subject to interpersonal power dynamics. This includes the charismatic power that accrues to certain teachers and some organisers. Part of that charisma is born from the evi-dent difference in who they are as a result of being remade by practice. As I will demonstrate later, the echoes of those domesticated experiences confer resonant charisma to the way they share practice, while the com-munity networks described here guard against any single teacher coming to dominate the subculture.

Whether charismatic teachers or not, all the organisers also maintain close relationships with those practitioners who are the most committed to other forms of activism. The mundane but significant personal sacrifice involved in organising an event is seen to be of a kind with the sacrifice involved in organising activist projects. And that activism encourages a much more pragmatic than charismatic self-presentation.

Not everyone in post-lineage yoga communities will be directly engaged in the higher-risk actions of environmental and social justice. But many post-lineage practitioners are in more supportive roles to action, gathering winter clothes to send to refugees in Calais, hosting fundraising events or joining communications blockades and boycotts. Of those that go further, some will do so because their own histories mean they are more comfortable with the social marginalisation involved, or with the scale of the task, and others because they are leveraging specific privileges to mitigate the risks.

The One Spirit Ashram Kitchen relies on all of these. In 2015, at the end of one event, two newly qualified One Spirit interfaith ministers were having a conversation about ministry:

> And there's a standard ministry with a capital M. Somebody doing funerals and weddings and baby naming, [and] [...] I said, 'Well, the Santosa kitchen's coming down today. We could take it to Calais and just do the kitchen.'
>
> (Ian, One Spirit Ashram Kitchen)

During the ongoing European migrant crisis, in 2015 the 'Calais Jungle' emerged as one of a number of unsanctioned refugee camps along the Northern French coast (Mould 2017: 3). Forceful policing by authorities and a lawless reputation meant few NGOs had any presence in such camps, but ad-hoc and independent activist groups were involved in various charitable endeavours there. The One Spirit Ashram Kitchen was one of these. Inspired by a religious instruction to serve, using the equipment from yoga community events, they used the knowledge of how to feed thousands for very little gathered in yoga event communal kitchens and Sikh *gurdwaras*.

> Just knowing how little it costs to serve per meal. [...] We came with that knowledge. And also, of everyone mucking in, what a great community thing it was.
>
> (Ian)

Those such as Ian, underwriting and overseeing the investment of infrastructure, had a little time and money to spare. And they were joined by a backbone of long-term volunteers who themselves lived transient lifestyles. Many of them were marginalised New Age travellers who had settled in Southern Europe.

Within such environments as these, where the very existence of the refugee camp was a daily struggle, activists relied on personal resources of equanimity, compassion and moment-to-moment awareness often honed in self-care practices, but the chaotic situation on the ground now made practice more pragmatic.

> I used to do so much mediation and 45 minutes of *mantra*s every morning. I've fallen off that horse somehow. [...] Living on the road and living out the back of a transit, really. It hasn't helped.
>
> (Ian)

The pragmatic activist and the event organiser have thus both evolved their practice to aim for a life that is 'good enough' rather than exceptional and thus charismatic. Case study 3, Uma talks about singing her daily mantras to Hanuman while driving from workshop to event. Case study 1, Veronika practices her *yoganidrā* with her children at bedtime. The activist-practitioner is pragmatic precisely because the personal rewards of practice have become subordinate to, indeed inseparable from life off the yoga mat. Their practice evolves to train for self-resilience, equanimity, and empathic compassion, in the hope of constructing a 'good enough', ethical life. And they believe that even the simple self-nourishment offered to beginners at a post-lineage event can be a radical act in a culture that values consumption and production above all else. As one activist from the group Rising Up[3] (see www.facebook.com/RisingUpUK) said to me: 'I think that ability to grieve and keep your heart open and not close down, I suppose that's really what I think [is] yoga.'

Such social justice concerns are the invisible context behind many of the intentions and rewards of post-lineage yoga. Communities of practice such as this one emerge from disparate groups of modern postural yoga practitioners, coming together in the search of answers that their existing practice could not provide. The community solidarity and experimental methods they develop attracts other teacher-practitioners from lineages more open to collaborative knowledge. The emergent subculture works hard to provide accessible opportunities for more people to discover not just the benefits of the practice, but the importance of a reflexivity that turns out as well as inwards. While the practice may entail fraught

---

3 There is a significant and fascinating research project to be done in tracing the evolution of the activist group Compassionate Revolution, into the movement known as Rising Up, and then into the globalised activist network known as Extinction Rebellion.

negotiations with difficult histories, hope for both personal evolution and social justice is ever present.

THEORISING THE CONNECTIONS SUSTAINING POST-LINEAGE PEER NETWORKS

This subcultural network has long-lasting ties and an evolving history, and regular but intermittent proximity. Coming together in person at post-lineage events is supplemented by more frequent interpersonal communication and promotional messaging online. Post-lineage yoga is a network, but the personal narratives and community solidarity that Wittel argues are absent from networked sociality (2001: 51–2) are in fact commonly shared here. This is not a bureaucratic database, but an informal flock, and not a managed hierarchy, but a loose network of friendships and working collaborations (Wittel 2001: 69; Lionel and Le Grange 2011: 745).

As Joost van Loon writes, 'Networks problematize boundaries and centrality but intensify our ability to think in terms of flows and simultaneity' (2006: 307). Affinity and charisma developed through post-lineage community interactions and shared narratives flows through and shapes its networks. Key figures in the network can be determined from their number of significant engagements with others (Adams 2013: 326). Charismatic, well-liked and well-connected individuals are disproportionately responsible for the norms shared here. But because post-lineage networks function with multiple points of feedback and reflection, they multiply the numbers involved in subcultural creation, preferencing collective processes of learning and evolution (van Loon 2006: 309). In the post-lineage environment, where practice is often shared by multiple bodies with multiple other bodies, the subculture evolves in a real time example of a gift economy, or more accurately, a *sevā* economy (Carrier 1991: 124).

Taking one example extracted from that data, and adding in known affiliations to groups, in Figure 3.3 can be seen the diversity of connections held by Uma and her partner Nirlipta alone. The resulting social capital is used to sustain and evolve Santosa year by year (Caldarelli and Catanzaro 2012: 31).

Among the most resilient social networks are those in which a small number of highly connected figures hold multiple connections with each other, and a much larger number of connections to the more weakly connected wider population of members (Caldarelli and Catanzaro 2012: 55). In network theory terms, the charisma that helps to attract a larger number

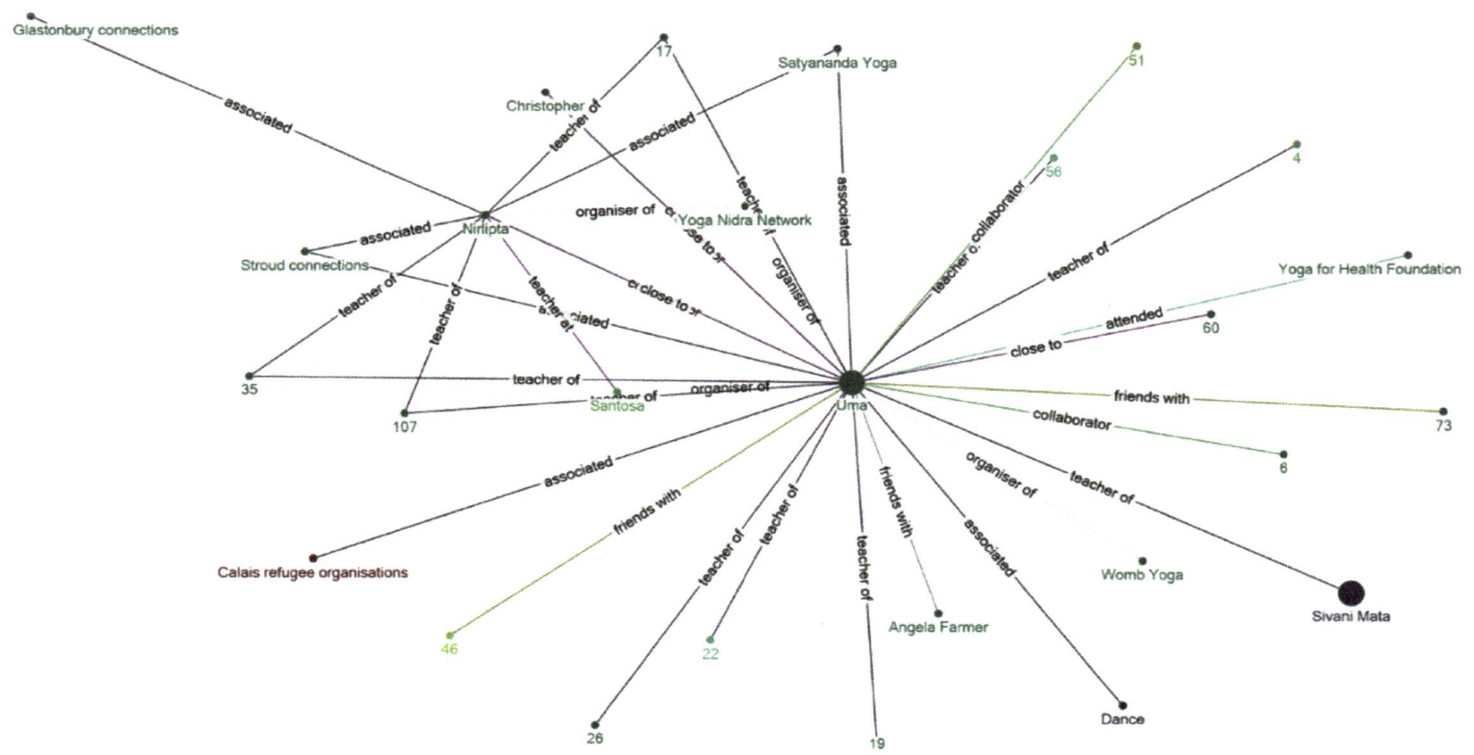

Figure 3.3
Networks: Uma and Nirlipta's alliances

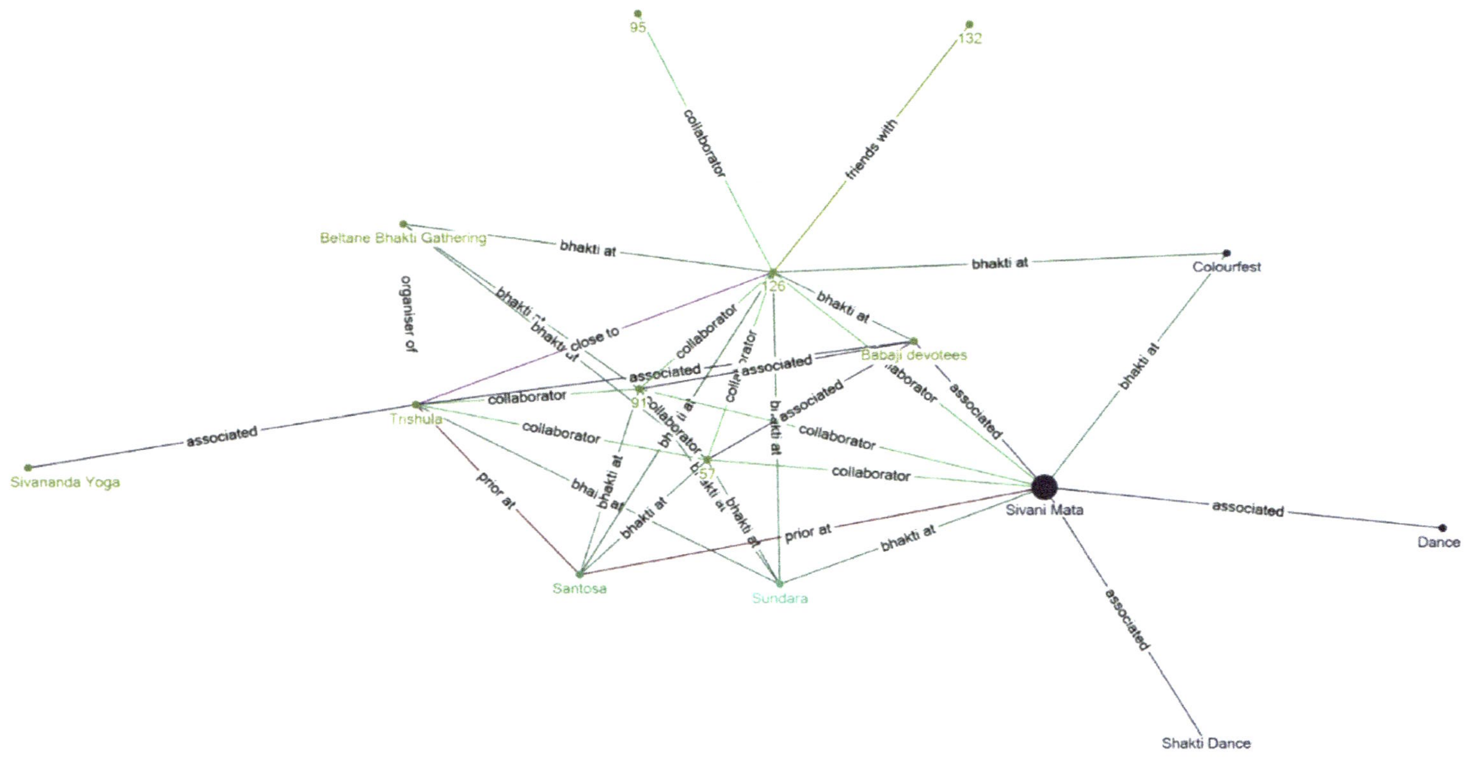

Figure 3.4

Networks: The Babaji Temple Singers

of more superficial connections to a few central figures with deeper connections to each other, can be understood as a measure of preferential attachment (Caldarelli and Catanzaro 2012: 71).

The shifting membership of the Babaji Temple Singers (Figure 3.4), functions as another such network in miniature. Unlike many lineage communities, their connections are as commonly made to those outside their lineage as within it. As a result of this willingness to connect, multiple members will work at many post-lineage events, but they do not rely on every member being present to perform.

These diagrams give some sense of the complexity of affiliations that influence the diversity of post-lineage subcultures. From Babaji devotees to Calais refugee organisations, and from Special Needs Yoga to **Shakti Dance**,[4] each of the affiliations adds their own flavour as they add to both practices and subcultural norms. As membership in this community evolves, so too does subcultural practice. A significant body of network theory suggests that this evolution is at the very least constrained by, if not wholly incompatible with the kinds of managerial standardisation and hierarchical organisation typical of brand and lineage knowledge production, which aim to preserve and propagate rather than evolve and diversify practice (van Loon 2006: 313). It is no coincidence that one of the most resistant subcultures to standardisation in contemporary yoga sustains rapid evolution and high levels of diversity. It is also one of the most resistant to commercialisation. Commercial entities from clothing companies to marketing applications undermine the rhizomatic integrity of the post-lineage subculture (van Loon 2006: 313).

CONNECTING TO A MORE THAN HUMAN WORLD

Besides the move from the universal to the particular, and from the teacher as central authority to the agency of the individual student, post-lineage yoga, at least in this subculture, is characterised by individualisation, pragmatism, and an engagement with the world that embraces messy and even uncomfortable edges. Although much yoga practice of any kind takes place in spaces that are pragmatically available, the ideal ecology of post-lineage practice differs greatly from the minimalist aesthetic of most

---

4 A Kundalini Yoga inspired combination of yoga and dance commonly taught at these events

contemporary yoga studios, which aim to separate the practice from mundane and chaotic reality (Thompson and Gates 2014: 68). In contrast, at post-lineage events the very ground beneath the practice is made smooth by the passage of feet. Practices of all kinds change with the weather and other environmental conditions. Practitioners snuggle into blankets during misty dawn meditations, crowd under canvas to share meals on rainy days, and during prolonged sunshine, some scatter for a little discrete naked sunbathing.

This is ecology with agency. It can be mundane and depleting, challenging and resistant, or humbling and nourishing. Every movement is a tactile relationship and a renegotiation with gravity, every meditative moment is an exploration of inside and outside and edges (Ingold 2011: 24). The body becomes that which one yoga thinker describes as a 'field of radiant sensation' (Miller and Schoomaker 2015: 183). We are, as Christopher will describe in Case study 2, a microbial temple. Every interpersonal connection in the subculture is embedded not just in a more than human ecology, but also in physical processes that post-lineage yoga practice variously enhances, and helps to render visible: mimesis, entrainment, and pheromonal attraction (Sheets-Johnstone 2012: 397). Any redrawn boundaries around the ideas of 'self' 'group' and 'world' that result can only be temporary.

Event organisers engage with the pragmatism of lived experience to differing degrees. Rowan at Colourfest wants participants to be comfortable enough to engage in the processes of discovery on offer:

> I've been to yoga festivals where it's been cold, wet, windy [...] and the capacity to grow and learn in that environment is more difficult [...]. So, we're trying to create an environment that's going to be optimum for that system to thrive.
>
> (Rowan)

While in the Santosa environment, Uma hopes that the process of meeting the basic needs of the physical self becomes *more* evident, encouraging self-reflection in a different way:

> You want a hot shower? There's the fire. I think it brings us back to what's absolutely real, that we have to get away from where you just have to turn the tap on.
>
> (Uma)

Their solutions may differ, but both start from the premise that lived experience is the ground of the practices they are promoting. And the embedded, embodied nature of this post-lineage subculture complicates any standardisation of the practice across a diversity of possible practice ecologies.

The named methods of practice that are taught here are rarely yoga brands or schools in the conventional sense. Labels are more usually used to signal whether a session offered on a schedule will be more challenging or less, or based on a specific ontology or epistemology. Thus, 'Chi Yoga' is so-named to signal its flowing and gentle approach, and '**Womb Yoga**'[5] to signal its adherence to divine feminine ontologies. Other teachers will use more generic names for their offerings on a schedule, and when asked, explain their teaching style by listing a blend of different influences that signal common subcultural reference points.

In a similar way, each event uses subcultural signifiers to signal its own unique flavour and contribution to the post-lineage community that moves from camp to festival. The most casual of attendees might only be aware of one post-lineage event, but the committed community member is conscious of an evolving calendar that fills each British summer. Some events will only last a weekend, others a week or more. There are overlaps and scheduling conflicts, regular commitments, fallow years, and one-off events. Those at the heart of the subculture will also need to schedule preparatory working parties, meetings, admin and marketing. These too are opportunities to come together with close friends and allies. Events are dreamt of in the winter, announced and planned each spring. Then each practitioner's summer is a unique and semi-nomadic journey from event to event, place to place, the *saṃgha* reforming again and again, returning home more or less often to rest, recover and earn money, then coming together once more.

---

5 Contemporary yoga school emphasising seasonal rhythms and the divine feminine developed by Uma Dinsmore-Tuli (Case study 3).

4

Yoga camp life

Most of the contemporary alternative yoga practitioners that I have met maintain an intense antipathy to large, mainstream yoga events such as the Om Yoga Show in London and Manchester (see www.omyogashow. com). They are considered to be an unfortunate, largely inaccessible but necessary evil at best, and at worst, emblematic of all that is wrong with mainstream yoga. Even the larger 'alternative' outdoor festivals, such as Glastonbury or Boomtown (Consultancy.uk 2017), are events that this post-lineage community attends with a mission in mind: to mitigate the hedonism, offer pastoral and holistic care, or help with the clean-up, recycling and re-purposing of festival waste. The camps and festivals that this subculture considers to be 'home', are smaller, less visible, and have a rather different feel and ethos. This chapter introduces just three of them, from an entire British summer of events: Colourfest, Santosa, and Sundara. It is followed by an overview of the themes and processes that characterise this subculture: common repertoires of practice; relationships with a more than human world; negotiations with lineage and ontology, and service as a form of yoga itself.

COLOURFEST

Our background is yoga but this festival opens itself to other ways to experience beauty and depth in life, whether it's through yoga, music, art, dance, storytelling, poetry or theatre.

(Rowan and Robbie, organisers of Colourfest)

The elegance of Colourfest's logo and high-quality photography of its website are reflected in the event itself, where white marquees seem to float in the landscaped grounds of Dorset country houses. In 2017,

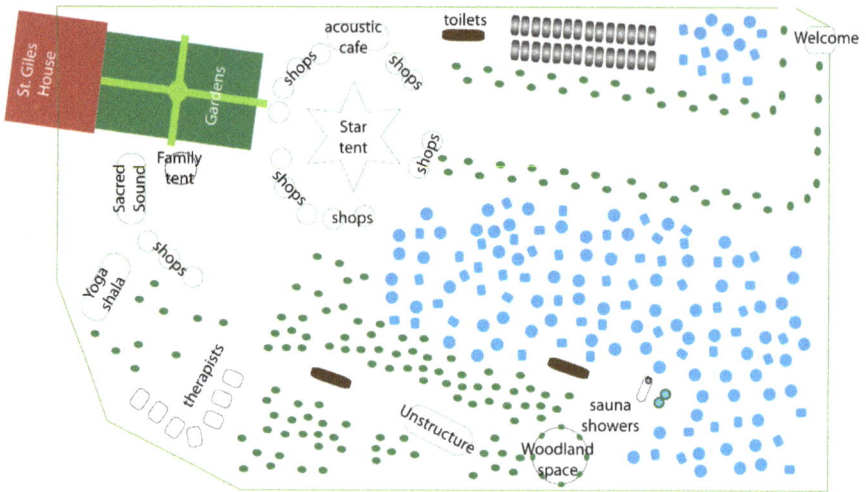

Figure 4.1
Map of Colourfest at St Giles House

Colourfest moved from its original location at St Giles to nearby Gaunts House. On both sites, as attendees, teachers and crew pick their way around the site, a sense of borrowed privilege is inherent in the feel of close-cropped lawns underfoot. Some of the sessions on yogic philosophy take place in libraries lined with leather-bound books. There are DJs playing in the evenings, under twinkling lights in woodland.

> Each year we get tighter. The flow of it gets tighter, the professionalism gets tighter. The beauty of the structures gets tighter.
>
> (Rowan)

It would be wrong to mistake the professionalism of the event that Rowan describes for commercial intent, however. Colourfest is not officially a non-profit organisation, but thus far it has aimed to break even on a £30,000–40,000 annual investment. A ticket to Colourfest costs around £150, but as many as a third of the people onsite will be working instead of paying for a ticket. The number of volunteers can be approximate, as people drop in and out up to the last minute, and none of the organisers of this or similar events collect exact demographical information about their attendees. But in general, there are around 1,500 people onsite during the peak weekend days. The organisers describe Colourfest as a 'festival', situating it with reference to similar events that are themed around music, art or dance. Attendees are more likely to be 20–50 years old, and a little more likely to be white, than the general British population.

Colourfest helps to cover its costs through licensing stallholders. In one area, there is a circle of such stalls selling clothing and a range of exclusively vegetarian foods, raw chocolate and turmeric lattes. Elsewhere on site is a canvas and wood burner, pay-for sauna. In various corners there are people playing with hula hoops and exploring partner acrobatics, as well as dedicated spaces for taught sessions of movement and stillness. This is a festival that appeals to a wealthy urban clientele, while also being tailored to the ethics, interpersonal interactions and consumption habits of yoga practitioners. Here they sell branded water bottles, and sport lotus flower tattoos.

The event's founders as well as organisers are two yoga teachers from Bournemouth:

> We started saying, wouldn't it be amazing if all the things we loved were in a festival?
>
> (Robbie)

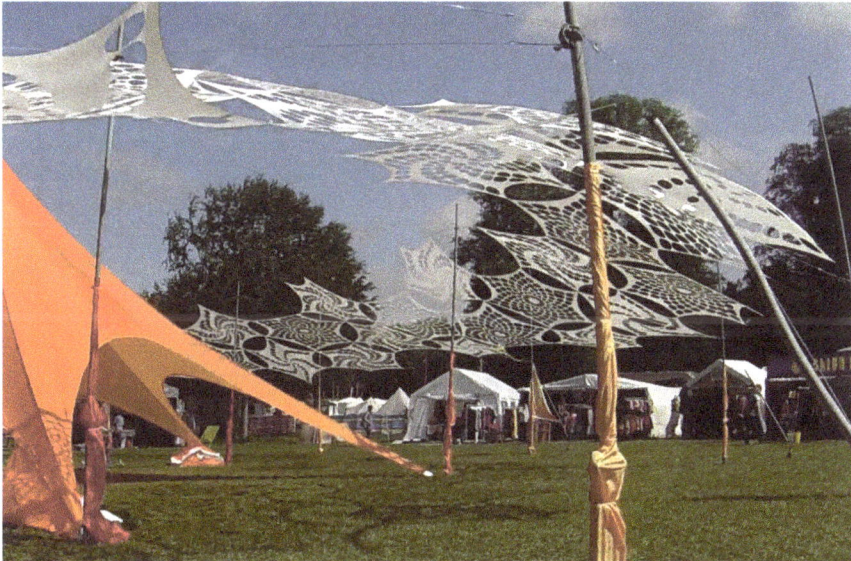

Figure 4.2
Colourfest at St Giles House (1)

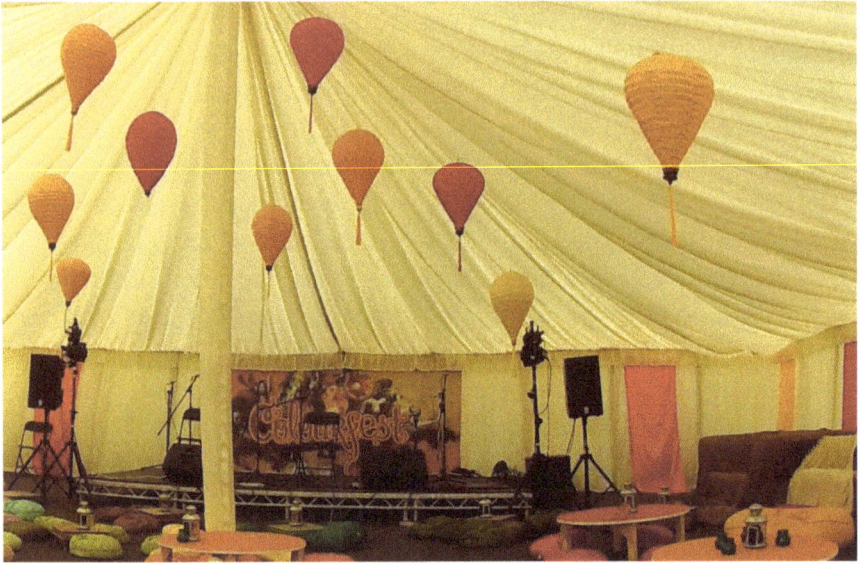

Figure 4.3
Colourfest at St Giles House (2)

Colourfest demonstrates the clear influence of rave culture on British yoga in its décor, music and the personal histories of many attendees. Yet the hedonistic substance usage that defined rave culture is categorically banned.

> I'd been [...] very disillusioned and disheartened by what I saw [at other festivals]. In the name of coming together I just saw disconnected debauchery.
>
> (Rowan)

A promotional film for the event describes Colourfest as 'a chance to deepen your own journey'. This is a festival as reimagined through the lens of contemporary yoga: less hedonistic, more athletic, delighting in interpersonal connection and promoting holistic self-development. Robbie and Rowan trained within the **Integral Yoga** lineage, developed from the teachings of Swami Satchidananda, so Colourfest's offerings are structured in accordance with the Swami's typology of yoga, which covers meditation, physical practice, devotion, selfless action, self-inquiry and *mantra* repetition (chanting).

Yet the yoga on offer at Colourfest is influenced by a diversity of schools and lineages. And beyond the early morning and evening chanting, silent meditation, and acrobatically sequenced *āsana* sessions accompanied by urban beats, there are also non-yoga movement disciplines to try, from African Dance to Contact Improvisation (a contemporary movement practice exploring movement in relationship with others). One experimental dance session brings three yoga and movement teachers together with live musicians. Thirty to forty people move and rest in turn, alone, in couples, and in trios, as a resident poet frames the experience with improvised, hypnotic lines:

> Spirit takes us back to our burden of green tangled, crazy hope. And we are no longer safe. But we are dancing, and we are dancing, free and mad.
>
> (Dance Jam session, Colourfest)

Elsewhere, Shakti Dance teachers combine **Kundalini Yoga** *mantra*s (a yoga practice developed from the teachings of Yogi Bhajan), with scripted dance and yoga postures. At the end of one such session that I attended, I lay back and listened to a dulcimer playing, feeling as if the little part of the world I could see was blessed and I with it. Even so, I remained acutely aware of how transitory the experience was, and how dependent on my curated and cultivated surroundings.

Colourfest is, for many, a step away from festival hedonism without the overt seriousness of many yoga retreats. What smooths that step is the quality of its surroundings, and the talents of those who work the event. As at each of these events, supporting the public face of taught sessions and performances is a broad web of interpersonal intimacy that crosses any boundary of school or lineage. Most noticeably, there is a way of interacting at all of these events that is rarely experienced in commercial yoga spaces. It is in the warmth of the greetings between friends and strangers alike, and the care with which people treat each other. It is how people in the same subculture relate to each other when two of their markers for shared identity are taking responsibility for their wellbeing and common ethical references governing interpersonal relations. And it may have a long history, given this contemporary description by Rom Landau of the 1927 Theosophical Star Camp in the grounds of a Dutch castle:

> They generally abhor the idea of meat as violently as that of wine or tobacco; they look deep into your eyes when they talk to you; they have weakness for sandals, for clothes without any particular distinction of shape, [...] and such colours as mauve, bottle-green and purple.
>
> (Goldberg 2016b: 55)

Those teaching at and running Colourfest are not spiritual entrepreneurs of self-interested wellbeing (Bowman 2009: 166). They are experienced and respected teachers and practitioners without international brand recognition (Goldberg 2015). Some of the teachers lead more comfortable and conventional lives but others arrive in live-in vehicles, or supplant meagre incomes by selling a little jewellery gathered on travels in India and South America. This is probably just one stop for them in a semi-nomadic summer spent travelling from camp to retreat to festival, taking on a variety of roles and responsibilities.

At Colourfest, the mainstream meets the counterculture. Many of the ticket holders come looking for an enjoyable festival weekend that might offer something a little healthier, or because they want to explore a little more of what yoga can offer beyond their local classes. They might consider yoga as part of a self-described spiritual-but-not-religious identity, a chosen element from those afforded by income and urban living.

But what is on offer at Colourfest is created and embraced by the network of people at the heart of the event. They come here mostly to explore new inspirations and to connect with friends, although as we shall see, there are more discrete flows of power and charisma at play here. And they have a distinct and shared cultural identity separate from the more casual attendees who come to practise with them, even though they may be well-used to serving their needs.

SANTOSA LIVING YOGA AND BHAKTI CAMP

While Colourfest is early in the post-lineage summer season, Santosa takes place in late August, when the British summer is already fading. This is also the longest event, a ten-day intimate gathering described as a 'camp', not a festival. The aim is to explore the idea of *saṃtoṣa* within community: lexicalised as Santosa, and defined here as 'the happy acceptance of what is, just as it arises'. Santosa prides itself on its survival, running every summer since 2005. Santosa's numbers are unlikely to top 250, and the full ticket price is around £375, but this includes all meals, and far fewer opportunities to spend money than at Colourfest. There is a small chai shop, and anyone may lay down a blanket and display a little handmade jewellery or second-hand clothing for sale. At all three sites, a handful of therapists offering everything from reiki to massage provide paid-for treatments onsite, and contribute a percentage of earnings to the event.

Santosa's annual budget is around £24,000, and it has occasionally made a profit, but more often a loss which its founders, Uma (see Case study 3) and her partner Nirlipta, are happy to absorb. Almost two thirds of the people onsite will be working in some way for their attendance, making donations to help cover costs. Including food deliberately attracts more young families, and older attendees appreciate the wider range of less physically taxing activities. There are also more attendees here of South Asian origin than at Colourfest, reflecting a greater emphasis on Hindu devotional rituals. Yet in this corner meadow within sight of Glastonbury Tor I meet a significant number of the same people who lead sessions at Colourfest.

More obscure forms of yoga are welcomed here. There are also sessions exploring the energy patterns of sound, belly dancing workshops, and meditations with natural elements reminiscent of the 'Council of Beings', in which 'participants prepare by spending an hour or so apart from other humans seeking an empathetic immersion into "nature"' (Harvey 2006: 182). Figure 4.4, for example, is a notation extract from the 'cacao ceremony', in which movement instructions are framed to honour the natural world.

"Cacao Ceremony" with Keef W. Miles - Hanuman Temple, Santosa 10.30 - 12.15 pm Saturday 27th Aug 16

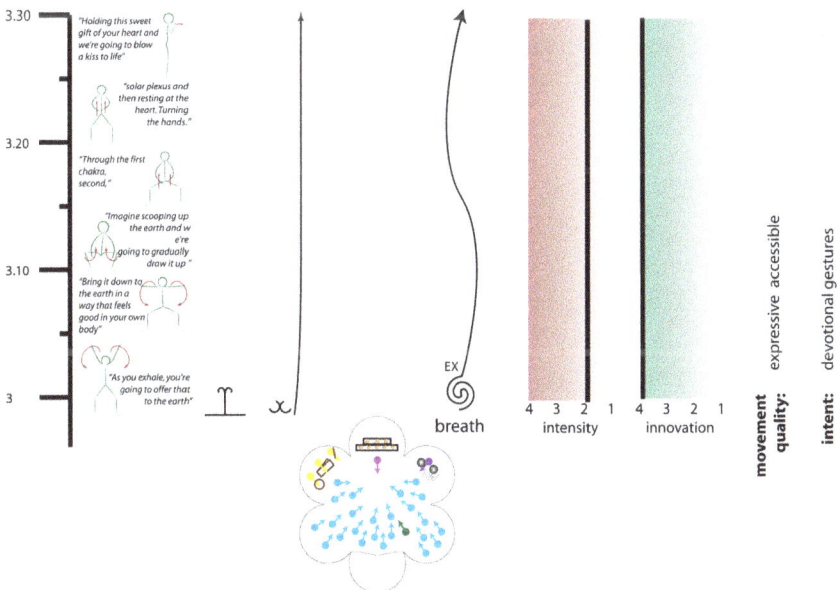

Figure 4.4
Santosa: Cacao Ceremony

There is a sense of experimentation here, using an intimate space among friends to explore new techniques together. This can rapidly expand everyone's personal and professional repertoire of moving, resting, or breathing. But from time to time the urge is strong for many long-term practitioners here to reconnect with their own movement habits. Solitary figures across the small site can be seen doing their established daily practice. Interestingly, a few teachers here and at other events will attend no peer-taught sessions at all. Once again, for them, the heart of the camp is in the making and maintaining of relationships with peers.

On-site, cars and live-in vehicles are segregated, but tents scatter and merge with the compost toilets, the communal field kitchen, the geodesic practice domes, and the interlocking nodes of the 'Bhakti Temple' yurt. Some low impact structures are up all year round. Others are dismantled and tucked away on site when not in use. Santosa grows each year from piles of canvas and wood, steel rigging, gas burners, and wood fired stoves.

Its layout is modelled on an imagined partial map of the yogic esoteric body. In the middle is the devotional temple space, seen as the heart centre of the site. Beyond it is the central fire, recalling the solar plexus. Beyond that is first the watery second *cakra* or energetic node, formed by the washing facilities, and then the earthy sacred grove, with its associations with the base *cakra*. It is commonly agreed that the site itself is particularly sacred, not only because of its sacred geometry, but due to the weight of years of repeated practice upon it, and its proximity to Glastonbury Tor.

Arising out of the edges of more mainstream yoga events, Santosa also has strong roots in the festival scene. The land is owned by the managers of Glastonbury festival's 'Healing Field', and as Uma describes it, Santosa was born from a familiar desire for the temporary autonomy and ecology of British festival spaces, bounded by contemporary yogic ethics:

> We'd had a really beautiful experience of being at the Yoga for Health Foundation which was in Ickwell Bury. But I never felt completely comfortable there [...]. We were the hippy, festie edge. And something in my little *yogī* soul was like: wouldn't it be nice if we could just let the kids run and there wouldn't be anyone who was off their head?

The camp began with little publicity, no budget, and no idea of how many people would come. Uma has attracted a revolving group of more practical people to help her, but the camp has kept to the same scale, same site,

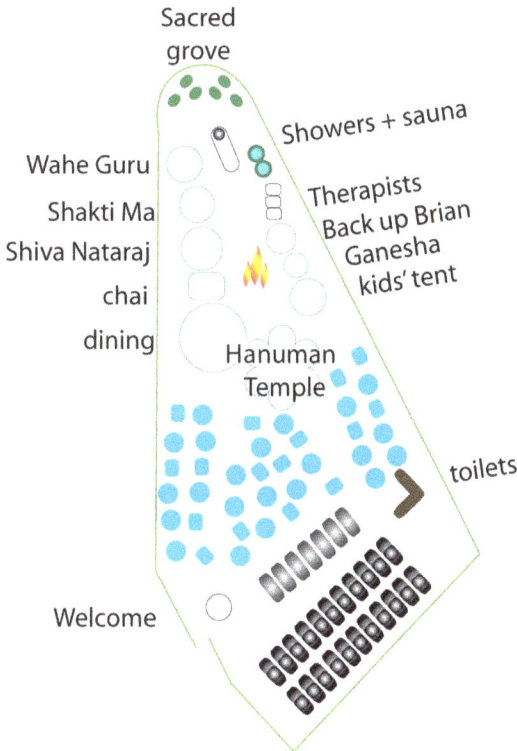

Sacred grove

Showers + sauna

Wahe Guru

Shakti Ma

Shiva Nataraj

chai

dining

Therapists

Back up Brian

Ganesha

kids' tent

Hanuman Temple

toilets

Welcome

Figure 4.5

Map of the Santosa site, near Glastonbury

and the same organisational premise, which Uma describes thus: 'It takes *tapas*, it takes disciplined effort, focused attention, [...] in order to create a situation where everybody can experience *saṃtoṣa*.'

Sustaining a yearly non-profit camp for over a decade is not easy. At any such event, a few key volunteers burn out or move on every few years. The interpersonal connections involved are more than just professional, and like any long-term community, romantic entanglements, family problems, and conflicts over finances and ethics can easily occur.

The terms Uma uses above, *saṃtoṣa* (ease) and *tapas* (discipline), are Sanskrit terms extracted from Patañjali's *Yogasūtra*, widely read by yoga teachers. With more yoga teachers in attendance, such conversational references to yogic philosophy are more common here than at Colourfest. Santosa is an event for those *already* trying to live an integrated yogic life. Time and again, yoga teachers talk of coming to Santosa as a form of self-sustenance. As Uma understands it: 'A lot of these people are teaching full schedules, from very authentic places, but it's very demanding, and they don't get paid a lot of money.'

This is an effortful form of communal sustainability, in which physical presence, simple service and constructive work are experienced as an essential form of nourishment that daily life and social media connections do not provide. My own experience of Santosa is marked by a productive tension between moments of ethnographic contemplation, and stepping into service. This balance of personal need and shared service is echoed in the organisation of the event itself:

> There's not a special VIP place for the teachers to park. [...] Everybody's at the same level. You know? The people who direct the camp are cleaning the toilets and chopping the onions.
>
> (Uma)

Above all, teachers are respected for their ability to teach to whoever arrives, and whatever the environmental conditions. Participants are encouraged to 'follow their own heart' and adapt the practices as they are taught here, but the land is an active partner in that process. At all these events, practice spaces are varyingly porous to dirt, weather, and the humans and other creatures passing through. And integration into Santosa's community is in part determined by how you interact with its most unconventional members. As one teacher says of one neurodivergent member: 'He's so fabulous, I adore that boy. He really triggers people, I love it. [He] is real, he can tell whether someone is bullshitting him or not.'

In part because of its longevity, of all three events Santosa is also the most consciously grounded in its ecology. There is nothing considered more appropriate in this context than muddy feet on a yoga mat. Even urine becomes a sacred offering to the land:

> Offering your liquid gold to the Mother. And to me that's a spiritual practice because it's like a reconnection.
>
> (Uma)

There is little artificial light on-site, and the schedule is constructed to synchronise visceral rhythms of activity, food and elimination, in the understanding that this increases interpersonal affinity. Outside of the more physical practice sessions, the core of the camp schedule is *bhaktiyoga*, which brings people's heart and breath rates into synchrony, and *yoganidrā*, which synchronises ultradian rhythms of rest. Within a day or so here, I take to wrapping myself in the softest of shawls and enjoy the daily rhythm of removing layers as the morning waxes, replacing them one by one as dusk slowly falls. An experience of Santosa is enchanted: both magical in feel, and grounded in the reality of weather, land, and bodies.

Community and interpersonal tensions, when they occur, are often expressed through the food on offer. Over the course of years there is an ongoing and covert, but friendly battle fought over the inclusion of eggs in the camp budget. In 2017 one volunteer left non-organic eggs from the local supermarket in the kitchen. By the next day, another had anonymously returned them. Everyone still eats together three times a day, with family, friends and strangers. As Uma writes: 'It was never about the money – it was always about sharing, and learning and practising together' (Dinsmore-Tuli 2013a)

SUNDARA COMMUNITY GATHERING

Balanced in the middle of summer, Sundara is the youngest of these events. Since its first year in 2015, numbers at the event are small, but growing. John and Tanya (see also Case study 5), the organisers, are in key roles at Colourfest, and spent a few years helping to run Santosa, and describe Sundara as a 'gathering'. Many of their teachers and crew are regulars at the other events and more besides. But the structures and location of the site for Sundara's first two years were dependent on another informal network rooted in British counterculture: the Rainbow Futures collective, who evolved from the camps of Rainbow Circle and Oak Dragon, which emerged in response to the establishment crackdown on travellers and free festivals of the 1980s (Worthington 2004).

As John told me, to put on an event like Sundara 'can cost anywhere between £15,000 and £20,000', and in these early years, they were still investing heavily in marquees, kitchen equipment and other infrastructure. A ticket for Sundara costs around £200 for five days. Interestingly, this means that all three events cost between £35 and £40 a day to attend, when paying full price. Again, all meals are included, and a chai shop, one or two stalls, and therapist commissions help to cover organisational costs. But here, as many as three quarters of attendees work for their ticket, paying slightly larger contributions than at Santosa to help cover costs. Together, there are around 250 people at Sundara during the peak

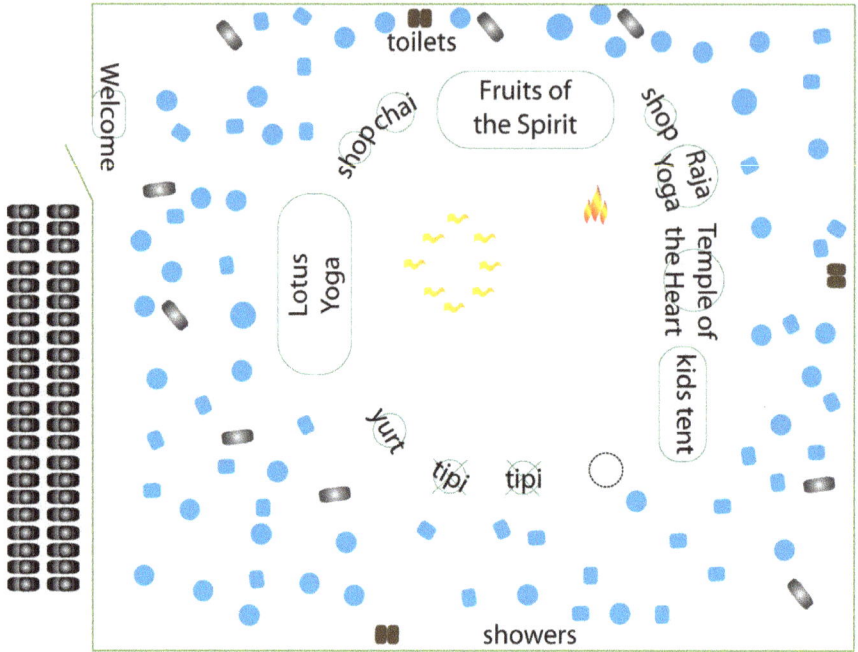

Figure 4.6
Map of Sundara on the Rainbow Futures site

weekend days. There is a relatively even spread of ages here, though not quite as many children and older people as at Santosa. Once more, there are also more attendees here of South Asian origin than at Colourfest.

The Rainbow Futures site that was home for the gathering for the first three years was a rented agricultural field atop a hill in the Forest of Dean, with the River Severn on three sides. More compact than either of Colourfest's sites, but larger and less contained by surrounding hedge lines than Santosa, it is approached via a long and narrow, winding road with discrete signage, and then up across a rutted field to flags flying on the windy hilltop. It was dotted with structures that Rainbow Futures would use throughout their summer of seven events, and then deconstruct and store for the winter, as sheep moved back in to graze. During my research time here, I witnessed the birth of a new community, as the seed of Sundara separated from Santosa, met the fertile ground of Rainbow Futures, and moved on again. Within the newness can be traced an inherited web of complex interpersonal affinities and tensions. After a divergence of aims with Uma at Santosa, John and Tanya had aimed to take a break from organising camps, but within a year, were running their own gathering, because, as Tanya put it, [the Rainbow site was 'literally on our doorstep, all the infrastructure is in. It feels like we've just been handed something on a plate'.

By 2018, they had moved again, on to another rented site nearby, and were constructing compost toilets with volunteers. They were encouraged and helped by many. The subculture as a whole is connected by mutual support and multiple opportunities to come together, and individual events are not competing for entrepreneurial advantage. As a result, a diversity of events signifies abundance rather than competition.

For Tanya and John, personal skills honed at raves and festivals, retreats and camps, as well as the interpersonal connections they afford, continue to be more valuable to the sustainability of Sundara than a frugal financial investment in infrastructure. Rather than relying on donations and serendipity, John says:

> I think an event can bounce along on the people that turn up and make it work for quite a while but if there isn't a definite financial plan [...] and organisation to it, eventually things start to degrade.

On both Sundara sites sat multiple canvas structures to house a diversity of practices, alongside wood-fired showers and sauna, a couple of stalls selling second hand clothes and original art, and a central fire circle. Regardless of the pre-published schedule, Sundara has a soft start, as does Santosa. A handful of people join in the first session of Dances of Universal Peace (a New Age group practice of dance and song). In one, a Buddhist *mantra* is sung with accompanying gestures of prayer in order to offer homage to *Buddha* (the enlightened one), *dharma* (spiritual path or teachings) and *saṃgha* (the spiritual community). By the start of the subsequent opening ritual, around 50 are usually present. Filling the schedule as numbers build to the weekend, will be another eclectic mix of dance, *āsana* and other movement sessions, meditations, relaxations and talks.

The food at Sundara is produced as part of a communal kitchen, like Santosa, here run by one of the main organisers of the Calais One Spirit Ashram Kitchen. Vegan stews and elaborate salads are supplemented by Tanya's own raw chocolate, on sale in the Chai Shop next door. 'Chai' is ubiquitous at these events, but unlike the highly sugared and caffeinated, Indian spiced tea that it is named after, this is adapted to the consumption habits of the community: sugar-free, and made with herbal Rooibos and plant milks.

Sundara is less earthy than Santosa, and less polished than Colourfest. Carpet is laid in many spaces. Practical service is optional but encouraged. The gathering also relies on a kind of low-tech cultural infrastructure that is common to the smaller events. Blackboards enable last-minute alterations to the schedule to be widely communicated. Conches are sounded or industrial-sized pan lids banged to mark the key moments of rituals and meals. At the daily morning meeting, the schedule is recapped, new arrivals welcomed, and any practical issues are shared. These innovations can be charmingly confusing to newcomers, even if they are yoga teachers, yet familiar to others who are used to attending similar countercultural events. They are rarely used at Colourfest, because the community that understands its norms is not in the majority there.

The yoga taught here at Sundara is both gentler and more unusual than at Colourfest, closer to that of Santosa, but with more sessions referencing Yogi Bhajan's Kundalini Yoga, reflecting the personal preferences of its organisers. Among the more eclectic sessions is Systemic Constellations, described as 'a mix of psychoanalysis, Zulu shamanism and phenomenology'. Most of the sessions have aims overtly related to personal transformation. One stalwart of the scene longs half-jokingly for a session of what he calls 'ordinary yoga'. There is one daily rest practice, often a gong bath (a guided sound healing practice). Like Colourfest, Sundara aims to offer multiple paths for self-development, but the ultimate framing is more communal:

> The idea is that people just come to a realisation that we can all actually live together happily. And do work on ourselves in a loving environment where other people are around.
>
> (John)

In its second year, the gathering's theme was 'Stepping up', with a focus on engaging in cultural change, inspired by the projects already started by key figures in the wider subculture:

> Well people are getting involved in things, [V] is off in the Amazon, Ian is in Calais doing the Ashram kitchen thing with [F].
>
> (John)

At Sundara teachers and crew are chosen for their ability to provoke transformation, as at Colourfest. They are prized for their commitment to certain norms of post-lineage yoga, as at Santosa. But some are also invited because they might inspire others to similar social justice projects.

In a quiet moment I visit a stone on the Rainbow Futures site that marks the spot where the man once known as the 'King of the Hippies' died (Worthington 2004: 46). His partner and a number of his children manage the Rainbow Futures camps in his memory, erratically supported by a chosen family of friends who raised children together at the anarchic Welsh land project known as Tipi Valley. In Britain, post-lineage yoga events are not only trading on the countercultural roots of British yoga, they are its continuation, involving many of the same people.

One possible interpretation of these three events would position Colourfest as bringing more mainstream yoga practitioners into easy contact with this post-lineage yoga subculture. Yoga, art and movement weave and meet at its many collaborative offerings. In the process, as elsewhere in contemporary yoga, *āsana*, meditation and dance become porous categories (Jacobs 2017: 4), in service to the larger aim of self-transformation. Santosa's community service is more inwardly focused. From *yoganidrās* to retellings of the origins of yoga, stories fill the space and mythologise the camp, and thus the subculture's own history. Santosa reassures people who feel on the edges of the communities they teach in that they are not alone, and that solidarity and a simpler, more sustainable, more sattvic (balanced) way of life is possible.

Within this reading, Sundara, the youngest of these three events, is a tribe of tribes, one meeting point in the semi-nomadic British festival summer. It brings together post-lineage practitioners with a number of other countercultural affinity groups. Of all the three, it is the most consciously built in the hope of better futures, with the labour of refugee activists and *bhakti* charities, from blueprints provided by traveller camps and intentional communities. If Colourfest bridges the mainstream with the post-lineage community, and Sundara links the same post-lineage community with the counterculture, Santosa is perhaps the most focused on serving this specific post-lineage community itself. And yet each of these descriptions can to a lesser extent be applied to the other events, and more events besides. They describe core processes and features that can be expected in any post-lineage subculture.

MOVING TOGETHER: COMMON FORMS OF PRACTICE

Any session at any post-lineage event can contain any combination of static postures, rhythmic movement, partner work, relaxation, contemplation, esoteric visualisation, chant and poetry. Each session is created from a half-hidden palimpsest of sources. One teacher at Santosa, for example, describes her teaching as a 'brew of Tantra with Scaravelli', but there are *āsana* postural sequences familiar from both the commonly taught Vinyasa Yoga (both a branded and generic term for movement-focused *āsana*, often set to music) and Uma's own Womb Yoga (see Glossary) in the session. In another relaxation session I recognise the distinctive phrase 'a radiant orb of sensation' from the American *yoganidrā* teacher, Richard Miller (2010), but only because I am familiar with his audio recordings.

The diversity of practice shared at these events prohibits a complete catalogue of its elements. Yet within this diverse repertoire, there are common bodily shapes, and some are allied to common intentions. Gestures of bowing are often associated with surrender. Gestures of opening and closing the arms and waves along the spine are often associated with breath and the heart, as seen in the dance session in Figure 4.7.

Movements that involve stepping and lunging are associated with change and willpower. These bodily shapes are common not just to *āsana* teaching, but also emerged as part of taught and spontaneous movements during *bhakti* and other communal activities. Taught *āsana* elements that are designed to provoke a challenge include balances, contorting the limbs, engaging the core muscles of the torso, repeated movements and

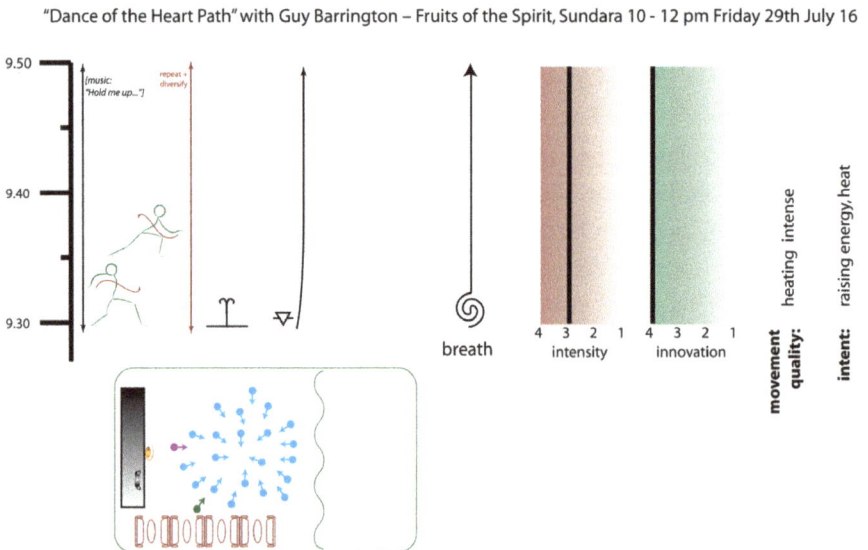

"Dance of the Heart Path" with Guy Barrington – Fruits of the Spirit, Sundara 10 - 12 pm Friday 29th July 16

Figure 4.7
Sundara: Opening and closing the arms

"The Beat Goes Ohm" with Natty and Scott - Yoga Shala space, Colourfest 7.30 - 9pm Saturday 4th June 16

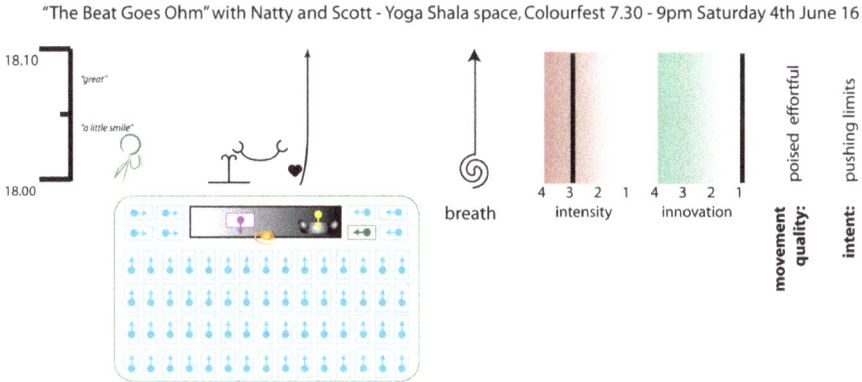

Figure 4.8
Colourfest: Smiling in squats

long holds. Challenging moves are experienced as more performative than contemplative, and likely to be accompanied by moments of shared humour, as when one teacher encourages participants to smile while the group holds a long squat, in Figure 4.8.

The instructions for each *āsana* may focus on specific body parts, most commonly the hands, feet, heart or spine. *Āsana*s may also be associated with specific muscles, joints, fascia, nerves or more esoteric features such as *nāḍī*s (energetic channels) or *cakra*s (major energetic nodes). More eclectic inspiration is found in the events' non-yoga offerings, and fragments from these find their way into many yoga sessions. Some hybrid forms are found on the schedules, such as the Shakti Dance sessions detailed previously, and Chi Yoga, which combines the flowing movements of yoga *vinyāsa* (moving) forms with more oscillating, back and forth movements from the Chinese practice of *qigong*. Each of these influences contributes to the *specific* practice repertoire of each individual, event, and subculture, but the *processes* of creating a shared, peer-dependent repertoire are more universal.

There is a shared language of and about movement, intention and bodily experience that has roots in more mainstream yoga practices. Typologies for describing a shared field of experiences are drawn from yogic and Ayurvedic categories based on the qualities of earth, water, fire, air and aether. But the repertoire this language describes diversifies rapidly here, and the typology enables newer and more obscure practices to be easily explained to others. Taught practices are also often described as more 'masculine' (effortful and directed) or 'feminine' (accepting and cyclical). One Shakti Dance teacher at Sundara describes the practice in 'feminine' terms of self-acceptance and cyclical rhythms:

> What we're doing is allowing the waves, the energetic waves within the physical form, within the energy body, within the mental body, to come into greater harmony and flow.

While another Shakti Dance teacher at Colourfest suggests a much more directed, 'masculine' intent: 'Hands like swords. Getting ready. You are focussing to cut your limitations, your attachments. Slow motion. Really sharp.'

Elsewhere, Santosa hosted a collaboration between two of my case studies: Uma and Christopher. The sessions were framed with reference to both Hindu and East Asian cosmology as a dance of 'Śiva' and 'Śakti', and the masculine 'yang' and feminine 'yin'. They contained some practices that toned the body and enervated the nervous system, others that encouraged rest and recovery, and some that investigated the boundaries between the two. The dance between 'masculine' and 'feminine', effort and acceptance, was embodied in the way Christopher and Uma responded to each other in their instructions:

> See how much you can press the shoulder blades down in the ground. How much energy can you create for a really substantial feeling of earthing through those shoulder blades and the back of the hands?
>
> (Christopher)

> [Your head] is just resting there. Let the earth carry your head.
>
> (Uma)

Most sessions taught at the events follow a wave of effort familiar from the evening *kīrtan*s (devotional singing, often in call and response form) led by *bhakti* singers: slowly rising in intensity before falling back into stillness. The ability to teach in this way enables shared peak experiences at the height of physical intensity, just as a DJ's choice of music enables the peak experiences of a rave.

In both taught sessions and individual practices, we find *āsana* postures from the Mysore lineages detailed in Singleton (2010), which have universally familiar names. Staying mostly within this repertoire allows teachers of the faster, more flowing forms to teach sequences without the need for extensive verbal instruction. It is assumed that each participant will know how to move into their appropriate version of downward-facing dog, for example. The teacher can then add more specific instructions. This is a methodology shared by many mainstream yoga events and classes, where a common if limited repertoire of practice is assumed.

Other postural shapes and sequences are variable signifiers dependent on each person's practice history. *Sūrya namaskāra* is a prostration sequence of early modern origin (Singleton 2010: 124), that almost all contemporary yoga students know. Beyond the basic postural waypoints, however, it has many variations. The intent behind practising any *āsana* can also differ, and the instruction that accompanies it may caution against anatomical alignments that another teacher might instruct as safe. Practice forms that embrace more unusual movements, further from the mainstream consensus, correspondingly spend more time on basic instruction, but are also likely to have unusual intentions. This includes the often-unique Kundalini Yoga **kriyā**s or cleansing practices.

The developers of more 'feminine' forms are wary of detailed direction entirely. These practices involve moving mostly in rhythmic circles and pulsations (see Sabatini and Heron 2006: 34). They are also more likely to be taught with the students and teacher together in a circle, rather than the teacher facing students that are arrayed in lines. The intent is to promote individualisation in movement, and so teachers suggest multiple options that defer to the authority of each person's needs. In one session of Scaravelli Inspired Yoga at Colourfest, the teacher instructs students to find their own practice variation to fit the experience that she wants them to have:

> You can come to more traditional movement. You can come to more animal-like movement. We're just playing with squats [and] that feeling of keeping our legs strong and our body light.

In reality, although it is possible to label many sessions as belonging to distinct schools, inspiration across school, intention and lineage is pervasive. There is no clear line to separate the movement repertoires and references of modern postural from post-lineage yoga. But what is definitional to post-lineage yoga as a whole is the prevalence of peer-based practice evolution, where teachers learn from each other, students are encouraged to individualise practice, and the roles of teacher and student are not permanently assigned, but lightly held in turn. The unsystematised, informal diversity and unique flavour of each post-lineage subculture arises from the many ways in which practice is shared unencumbered by lineage affiliation, teaching hierarchy, bureaucratic oversight or brand copyright.

CREATING SPACE: INNER AND OUTER ECOLOGIES

However it is taught, each yoga practice here happens in a specific space. As Sandra Sabatini, student of Vanda Scaravelli, writes: 'when standing, the spine moves and extends, between the ground below and the sky above, and the body fits into this dimension' (Sabatini and Heron 2006: 114). Every event organiser negotiates the compromises inherent in entering into landscapes marked by prior use. Colourfest must integrate into formal grounds without damaging landscaping. The shape of Sundara is dependent on the structures that they or their hosts can provide. Santosa is marked by its proximity to Glastonbury as a town and festival.

The events are bounded by time as well as space, crowding into the short British summer. Autumn and winter are dreaming seasons for the subculture, where little happens, and early spring marks the start of negotiations with the land and its gatekeepers. Unpredictable weather necessitates adaptation and thus diversity. Yoga sessions at the events are more likely to be vigorous when the weather is damp or cold, and escape their allotted canvas spaces to stretch on the grass when the sun shines, as in Uma and Christopher' session in Figure 4.9 and 4.10.

Practices with descriptions such as 'natural' or 'authentic movement' are scheduled into the wilder spaces at the edge of event locations. Santosa's emphasis on peer-to-peer networking is reflected in the non-hierarchical circularity of its canvas practice domes. Meanwhile, participants move fluidly from one space to another. They wander in and out of workshops that have been only briefly described. As timings slip and schedules evolve, they find themselves in practices they didn't so much choose as a consumer, but come across as explorers in an imperfectly mapped land.

The porousness of the canvas structures themselves means the content of each session slips osmotically into other spaces. At Nicole's Soma Yoga session at Colourfest (see also Case study 6), once the tent was full, people gathered outside to practise out of earshot, copying those closer in a kinetic version of a game of whispers (Figure 4.11). In a moment of serendipity, the sounds of the gong bath coming from the tent next door, provided a fitting substitute for those who could not hear Nicole's final relaxation instructions. Yet not all such crossovers are welcomed. Sessions

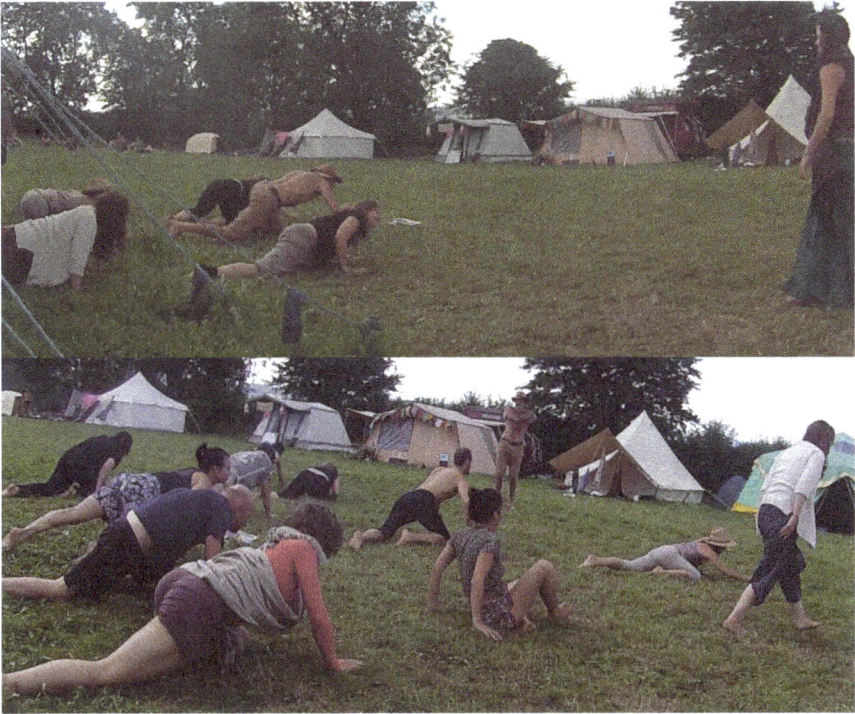

Figure 4.9
Santosa: Escaping boundaries

"Who Invented Yoga?" with Uma and Chris - [outside] Shiva Nataraj, Santosa 10.30 - 12.30 pm Monday 29th Aug 16

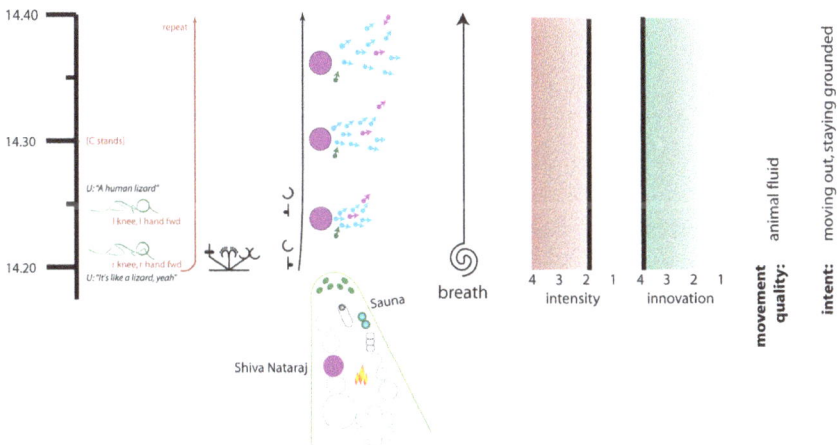

Figure 4.10
Santosa: Escaping boundaries

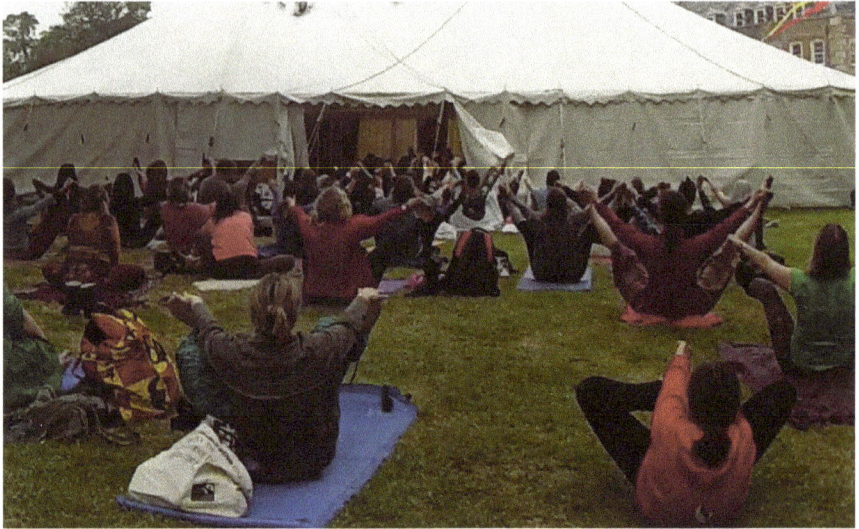

Figure 4.11
Colourfest: Teaching with osmosis

that include amplified music are openly challenged because of their tendency to bleed into others that involve contemplative stillness.

As porous and temporary as these practice spaces are, each mat, each structure, holds a long weight of history to those at the heart of the community. Their fragile, negotiated borders mark the boundaries of authority, of meaning, and of home. A post-lineage subculture that does not need to concentrate its communal activities into a few short months of the year might be more diffuse, and less coherent. One that shares its practice in more formal spaces might have clearer divisions between its composite affinity groups, and less serendipity in how each practitioner finds new sources of inspiration.

As Andrea Jain writes: 'a nondual metaphysics – a denial of the fundamental difference between the material world and the sacred world – characterizes postural yoga culture' more generally (2014a: 104). Within many sessions at these events, devotional content includes bodies mimicking and internalising the external ecology. Teachers and practitioners talk about the 'petals' or 'lotus' of the heart, the 'wings' of the arms and the 'roots' of fingers and toes reaching into the earth. Those *āsanas* with common names of natural origins become more extended metaphors. Practising *vṛkṣāsana* (tree pose) is a chance to explore the psychologised quality of rootedness involved in standing on one leg like a tree trunk.

This intimacy of ecology to practitioner is one I will return to. Here, where practice necessitates negotiating with the ground and everything that moves on or through it, the event community enacts and reinforces a shared relationship to the earth together. Over time, from Sundara to Colourfest to Santosa, each site is remade to reflect the enduring relationship between the landscape and its inhabitants (Johnson 2002: 305).

SHARING DEVOTION: NEGOTIATING LINEAGE AND BELIEF

Gurus whose lineages focus on *āsana* practices are much less likely to be a focus for allegiance here, although images of Yogi Bhajan (Kundalini Yoga) and Swami Satchidananda (Integral Yoga) in particular may be found on altars. Between Colourfest, Santosa and Sundara, other gurus that are celebrated include Sri Haidakhandi Babaji (one of numerous Hindu saints known as Babaji, as mentioned by Trishula previously), and Mata Amritanandamayi (one of several Hindu saints known as Amma). These lineages emphasise devotional service (*sevā*), humility and communal acts of worship over physical or meditational practice. Their devotees are more common in the ranks of volunteers than teachers, and thus offer service rather than knowledge transmission. This is not to say that these lineages are non-hierarchical, but those of their devotees who engage in post-lineage subcultures, are those who take their guru's injunction to serve humanity regardless of religious affiliation most to heart.

Overall, practitioners in this subculture are more likely than many to have had direct contact with 'the charismatic authority' of a living guru (Singleton and Goldberg 2013b: 5). But they are also more likely to take issue with the institutionalisation of authority in general. In all post-lineage subcultures, each person negotiates a unique journey of conforming to and questioning the norms that they receive from their teachers, and the wider culture. Lineage is one of numerous significant sources of inspiration, but those who are most convinced that lineage is the absolute authority over practice are least likely to be comfortable in any post-lineage environment.

Less well-known postural lineages also have a strong presence at these events, including Kundalini Yoga, which focuses on esoteric transformation through the medium of *mantra* and breath manipulation, as much as through *āsana*, Integral Yoga, which promotes a holistic, non-sectarian spiritual practice, and Yin Yoga, which uses long holds to release physical tension and psychological trauma, as well as the less structured, divine feminine schools inspired by the work of Vanda Scaravelli (1991) and Angela Farmer. Almost all the practices shared at post-lineage yoga events are accessible regardless of affiliation or experience, and a mutual respect for practitioners of other lineages or none at all is greatly encouraged. It is a prerequisite for those extra-lineage relationships on which post-lineage yoga is founded, and within which those who have rejected lineage entirely can find an equal welcome.

Within the community are many whose encounters with lineage and guru have ended badly, yet specific ethical breaches are rarely discussed unless they have recently become common subcultural knowledge. There is as yet, for example, little discussion of recent scholarship showing that the history of Kundalini Yoga differs greatly to the lineage's own narratives (Deslippe 2012: 371). Nor does the subculture openly discuss credible allegations of criminal activity by the founder of the lineage (Remski 2018a).

But during my fieldwork, a major investigation broke into sexual abuse within the **Satyananda Yoga** organisation, a lineage inspired by the teachings of Swami Satyananda (for details see Remski 2014a). These allegations *were* discussed, and the resulting shared grief was palpable among devotees and non-devotees alike, especially at Santosa. Satyananda Yoga is one of the main sources for the original development of modern *yoga-nidrā* (Birch and Hargreaves 2015b), leading to a public statement by Uma and her husband Nirlipta being added to their Yoga Nidra Network website (Dinsmore-Tuli and Tuli 2018c).

Beyond this specific subculture, and just as my research came to a close, allegations of sexual abuse by the founder of Ashtanga Yoga began to resurface after years of persistent rumours (Remski 2018b). As I will discuss in my concluding chapter, post-lineage connections and even hashtags have already influenced the public responses of at least some Ashtanga Yoga teachers within yoga-related social media spaces.

Devotees of all lineages and none thus practise together in post-lineage spaces. Continued adherence to lineage is rarely used to decide practice, but does create closer affinity groupings within the wider network, and so contributes to the specific flavour of individual events and even subcultures as a whole. In this, it is possible that the more outward-focused practices of devotional yoga lineages are an influential model for the changing nature of authority within post-lineage *āsana* practice. As one Babaji ritualist described it, the commitment that their devotees wish to inspire in others is not to a guru, but 'to truth, simplicity and love'. At Colourfest, Rowan publicly compares his relationship with Swami Satchidananda to the individual journey of each attendee who can explore 'your own way of reaching the silence ... the peace ... the heart'.

Within this specific subculture, the *person* of the guru is always absent, and any memory of the guru serves as a touchstone for a devotee's history of belonging to a supportive religious community. The devotional status of each guru may thus persist for some attendees, but regardless of any such affiliation, knowledge, ethical behaviour and emotional support are still disseminated through each wider post-lineage community on a peer-to-peer basis.

Some scholars claim that for contemporary yoga practitioners, the healthy body is the only goal (Jain 2014a: 62), and yet emic accounts of contemporary yoga often make such statements as: 'if we dedicate ourselves to practice, it is only a matter of time until the mat becomes an altar' (Cope 1999: 269). Without a baseline of evidence to measure from, it is unclear whether post-lineage yoga is inherently more or less religious in its intentions than either commercial brands or orthodox approaches to lineage, even if a metric for such religiosity could be agreed. But logically, we might expect a comparative survey of post-lineage subcultures to demonstrate a diversity in the levels of devotional intent, equivalent to the diversity of practice itself.

Within this subculture, each of these events do contain overtly religious content. Their sites are constantly being remade as sacred by the movement of people within them (Miles-Watson 2016: 39). At Colourfest and Sundara there are altars in teaching and performance spaces, while Santosa's Bhakti Temple is a multi-lobed yurt at the heart of the site, in which can be found, as Uma describes it, 'this amazing altar with everything that anyone thinks is holy is welcome up there.' These altars contain multiple **mūrti**s (divine representations) in the form of statues and images. As in traditional Hinduism, *mūrti*s are considered to be living incarnations of deities and gurus, with agency and needs. At Santosa, they are washed, anointed and fed daily, before taking their place among objects of natural beauty. The relationship between self and *mūrti* here is a complex one, in which the actions of cleansing and offering nourishment reflect the inherent non-dual divinity of all matter, including the body of the devotee. Individual participants may diverge from that metaphysical understanding of such ritual acts, but the widespread inclusion of *mūrti*s on altars confirms their centrality to devotional life here.

Pūjās that include more substantial offerings to *mūrtis* may happen once or twice during each event, but the devotional singing practices called *kīrtans* are scheduled multiple times a day, and many ritualists are also devotional or *bhakti* musicians. As elsewhere, *kīrtan* here is a populist religious practice, one that is 'improvised and situational' (Orsi 2012: 151–2). It moves through a rising tempo of repetition into a hypnotic and ecstatic liminal state often described as 'heart-opening'. The *kīrtan* chants are created through the lyrical, often call and response repetition of the names of divine beings (Pettit 2014: 14). This practice of naming as honouring is echoed at the smaller events with open morning meetings, in which each person present is also greeted by name and a '*namaste*'. This daily community ritual is even referred to as 'reciting the holy names'. All these devotional attitudes: to land, to people, to diverse representations of the divine, serve to enhance and honour the connections between them, and to apply a shareable vocabulary to the intimate ontologies that are explored in individual practice.

There are significant differences within religious content however. At Colourfest, religious references and communal practices tend to have more neo-Vedāntic content, bringing in revered teachers to give lectures to attendees. At Sundara, where the content of sessions is the most eclectic, inspired by more (core) shamanic and New Age practices, teachers assume a familiarity with crystals and other New Age epistemologies. And at Santosa, the practices on offer include more European pagan, but also more Tantric references. Key figures who attend Santosa work more or less directly with historic source texts. A number of them can read Sanskrit to some level.

Although these are communal religious activities and discussions, the specific ontological orientations of individuals are frequently obscured in public speech. A multiplicity of Hindu, Buddhist and pagan gods, gurus, saints and *bodhisattvas* are involved in morality references, mythological story-telling, *kīrtan* invocation and ritual *pūjās*. But these are placeholder terms for what are often private metaphysical attitudes. Glossing belief while continuing to involve the gods in worship and teaching allows participants to approach every figure on the altars as either a living deity, an incarnated natural force, an abstracted human concept or an aspect of a single god. But those attendees whose practice does not include devotion of any kind can feel marginalised. Nonetheless, the overall religious attitude of this subculture is henotheistic: accepting of other deities and concepts of god while retaining personal devotional allegiances.

In Britain at least, the extra-lineage activity undertaken by devotional subgroups at the events, such as the devotees of Babaji and Amma mentioned above, may be specific to those Hindu communities whose members are mostly white rather than diasporic, although the work of Maya Warrier demonstrates that such groups are also favoured by the Indian middle classes (Warrier 2003: 214). The overt syncretism of post-lineage yoga partially guards against many universalised narratives, including ethnic and religious nationalism. But issues of race and ethnicity are not absent from this or any (sub)culture. Religious expression is both constrained by, and constrains, all 'terrestrial, corporeal, and cosmic' transformations from one cultural reality to another (Tweed 2006: 75). Speaking of her own Indian heritage, Trishula (organiser of the Beltane Bhakti Gathering) told me:

> The irony is that I came back to it through westerners, through people whose lineage it wasn't because maybe they had fresh eyes, they had an innocence, they had a new love for it.

OFFERING SERVICE: BUILDING COMMUNITIES

Those attendees who are uncomfortable with *bhakti* practices at these events still engage in communal religious practices, through the shared work practices known as *karmayoga* or *sevā*. *Sevā* is perhaps the most important and universal moral value of this post-lineage subculture. Originally, *sevā* narrowly denoted the practice of service to deity, guru and devotees, but 'in its modern sense of organised service to humanity, [it] has become a marked feature of an increasing number of recent and contemporary Hindu movements since the mid-19th century' (Beckerlegge 2015: 39), and '*sevā* is a highly portable religious practice' (Beckerlegge 2015: 53). In this subculture, it is a way to perform community values of service and humility at the events themselves, and enact them upon the wider community, in charitable works and community service. As Trishula's husband says during a ritual at Colourfest:

> It's the easiest form of yoga. Everybody can do it. Not much excuse to not be able to serve, really. [...] Don't wait to be asked. Yeah, it's a very, very fast way to purify your mind and your heart.

Sevā fulfils a number of connected functions to support the community and its values, in ways that appear to be significantly different to the politically astute, organised social programmes associated with large Indian lineages (Beckerlegge 2015: 210) and the self-promotional, competitive charity drives of brand-based organisations (Koch 2015: 73). At every event the payment in kind represented by *sevā*, undertaken by organisers as well as teachers and crew, is a significant contributor to financial and community stability. Shared work reinforces communal solidarity (Wenger 1999: 78). But it also overtly encourages the do-it-yourself aspect of temporarily autonomous spaces, and thus aligns these events with countercultural values such as personal accountability, ecological frugality, and communal inter-dependence. At Santosa, having to commit to *sevā* in advance is even discussed as a useful screening process for attendees that do not share the community's norms.

Trishula makes a deliberate axiological connection between service and spiritual development that is a rejection of hedonistic self-interest. As she put it: 'Ram Dass puts it beautifully he says "It's about being free not being high and there is a difference."'

There are many within post-lineage yoga who, as she does, claim indifference to the very modest financial rewards involved. These are events where the organisers' reward is not quantifiable as a growth in income or commercial visibility. The mechanisms of financial exchange and brand coherence involved in running them are a symptom of their socio-political embeddedness within neoliberal capitalism, but do not negate their attempt to resist it. Personal and shared landscapes of land, gods and gurus, as well as alternative networks of value and exchange, become apparent when we look deeper than the immediate socio-political context to consider the motives and agency of those involved (Kraft 2002: 172). And far from operating according to the values of the casual consumer (Urban 2000: 296), the alternative exchange mechanisms in play here are carefully evolved and mutually negotiated.

Within the research, some respondents have used the term radical to describe this subculture. As Uma says when discussing Santosa: 'I love the word radical, because it's about, right down deep at the roots of people's lives and ways of living, something is being nourished.'

But part of the radical difference of post-lineage subcultures from the perceived traditions of yoga involves more horizontal status structures. And therefore, because radical and conventional are terms defined qualitatively and relationally, some participants find such terms divisive:

So, I don't feel that we're radical, we're not trying to push up against anyone, we're not trying to prove something to someone. [...] We're not pushing, we're not providing it as 'We know the way in, you're all lost if you're doing that and we know the way in, come and join this.'

(Rowan)

And yet post-lineage practice, at least for this subculture, takes place in some very unconventional spaces. Many of my respondents felt more comfortable with political activists than with what they often called the 'capitalist yoga scene'. The crossover between activist and yoga communities, in membership and in behavioural norms, seems to be increasing. Some within the post-lineage subculture had their lives changed as a result of volunteering for projects such as the One Spirit Ashram Kitchen in Calais, returning to set up yoga programs to support vulnerable populations in their home towns. For other post-lineage yoga teachers, the urge to help refugees came of watching migrants washed ashore at European retreat centres. Many contemporary yoga teachers are aware of the ongoing refugee crisis without being moved to get involved. An established yoga practice is not a prerequisite for thriving in activist environments. But the habits and practices of the post-lineage counterculture does support significant numbers of yoga practitioners in their activism:

And whether that gives you on the inside some inner strength to drop the importance of possessions, or [...] to take the risks. To take the gambles.

(Ian)

For Ian, what bound them together: organisers, volunteers, and refugees, yoga practitioners and not, is a shared experience of finding community in marginalisation:

It's people living outside of the system. Or people pushing the barriers and having the imagination and the strength to think it doesn't have to be like this, it could be like this.

A UNIQUE SUBCULTURE EVOLVING THROUGH COMMON PROCESSES

Post-lineage yoga may be practised in many more places and ways than we might yet know. But here it is both enabled by, and creative of, the distinct subculture of its summer events. These events are where the mainstream meets one edge of a surviving countercultural community, and where borrowed privilege meets social justice in the common dream of a hedonistic festival reimagined. At its heart stand key individuals, whose practices and inter-relationships this book will turn to next.

Simple service and a valorisation of natural rhythms combine to nourish a community of teachers from many lineages and none. The practices they share show evidence of a palimpsest of sources, and oscillate between intentional transformation and nourishing self-acceptance. They teach in spaces that are porous to their ecology and osmotic to each other, as music, instruction, lineage and even community soften their borders to meet each other. They call the holy names of the community and engage in henotheistic, multi-denominational, but overtly religious rituals. It is probable that similar processes may be found wherever a post-lineage subculture is able to thrive.

In each post-lineage yoga subculture, the intricate web of inter- and intrapersonal connections is also marked by long histories, impersonal forces, divine influence and seductive pollutions. The subculture is formed on and nourished by the land and its inhabitants, shaped by history, animated by *prāṇa* (life force). While much of contemporary transnational yoga practice may indeed be confined to a physical practice and its physical benefits, within this post-lineage subculture at least, it is assumed that one's practice of yoga also includes ethical, interpersonal, ecological and, to a lesser extent, political engagement.

The yoga practice found here is diverse, but it centres on the common subcultural perception that neoliberal lifestyles have a polluting effect, which encounters with yoga practices and the natural environment can purify. This is evident not just in the preference for muddy feet on a mat, but also in ambivalence to commonly used smart phones and a suspicion of vaccines and contrails. Given yoga's eternal concern with health and wellbeing, it is unsurprising that all these technologies are accused of making us sick. For many post-lineage practitioners, our very bodies are being invaded and our minds seduced by neoliberalism, and the evidence is written on the sky above them (Crockford 2017: 178).

Beyond common conventions for interpersonal conduct, the levels of engagement with radical politics or ways of living here are dependent on personal affordances, as much as they are influenced by a subculture that carries the legacy of key British countercultural moments. This legacy is renewed as with each generation, more activists become involved in self-care communities in order to sustain their activism. Radicalism and orthodoxy in the practice form, teaching and cultural politics can inter-relate in many meaningful ways. Each session of post-lineage yoga is located somewhere on a spectrum of innovation from the normative to the improvised, and each teacher on a spectrum from those who maintain strong links to lineage, to those that reject it completely.

Over and again, post-lineage practitioners here speak of the place of balance and the seat of wisdom as being with the hands, at the heart. As one of my case studies writes:

> The heart-space has been seen as the gateway to trans-personal reality and real 'spiritual' identity (the post-rational divine) since ancient times.
>
> (Gladwell and Wender 2014: 59)

As we shall see in the next two chapters, this specific post-lineage sub-culture, as well as the processes that support its communal evolution and solidarity, depend also on the long-term, individual practices of its key members. It is in those practices that the relationship with the 'inner teacher' is born, and it is those practices that this book now turns to examine.

PART II

ON THE MAT

5
Case studies

INTRODUCTION

In Part II, we move away from the *interpersonal* towards the *intrapersonal* aspects of post-lineage yoga. Each of the following case studies was chosen as an example of thematic currents within this subculture, and each person is a key figure in the network. Each one demonstrates the diversity of individual practice, but also illustrates the common processes that underpin practice development. Every individual practice both contributes to and depends on the group norms of its specific subculture. As such, each one further illuminates the negotiations between adaptation and authority introduced in previous chapters.

Together they demonstrate a series of productive relationships. In the first case study, we see the tension between self-acceptance and the ideal self, and in the second, between resilience to the natural world, and the self as a microcosmic temple. The third case study demonstrates the internal dance of different elemental selves, and the fourth shows the use of ritual in the creation of self-intimacy. In the fifth, self-discipline is used to sustain the ethic of service, and in the last, sacred ceremony reveals the mysteries of inner landscapes. Taken as a whole, the case studies demonstrate the productive tension within each practitioner and thus the subculture as a whole, between lineage and peer authority, single and multiple voices of identity, and between the desire for self-acceptance and for self-transformation.

My understanding of the intention and lived experience of each co-practice is grounded in each respondent's own explanations to students in teaching situations, their own words in online and print media, and above all in the interviews that follow the co-practices. Unless otherwise referenced, in this chapter all direct citations come from the practitioners themselves.

Each of the case studies also represents a unique example of the co-practice moment. For each one, I meet each respondent in their own practice, follow them as best I can, and then interview them about their practice: its history, influences, and that day's manifestation. Although the modern history of yoga transmission relies on various forms of co-practice as bodies moving and sitting together, rarely is the individual practice of a practitioner given such undivided attention by a witness. Therefore, not only is this data unique for research into yoga, the method itself was a unique process for yoga as a practice. The experience of co-practice itself, beyond the data produced, reveals profound insights into the nature of shared practice that I will return to in later chapters.

CASE STUDY 1

The 'pristine body'

VERONIKA

I first met **Veronika** at Santosa, accompanied by her youngest children. At the age of 27, suffering from chronic pain, she had encountered her first experience of returning 'to a place where [the] body feels good'[1] in Sivananda Yoga classes. She went on to discover Ashtanga Yoga, trained to teach as an Ashtanga Yoga teacher, and continued to practise and teach according to that lineage for many years. Ashtanga Yoga teachers are not usually taught a practice of seated meditation, and Veronika's independently held belief that every yoga teacher should also know how to meditate led her to her first **Vipassana** course (for a description of this popular Buddhist form of meditation see Hart 2011): 'It totally blew my mind. [...] I practised every day. [...] I was becoming more equanimous, and more settled within myself.'

At this point she began combining practices from two lineages that each complemented the gaps she saw missing in the other. Her practice journey demonstrates the compromises practitioners typically make between dedication to the teachings of specific teachers, and a growing awareness of individualised needs that necessitate wider explorations in practice.

Veronika credits her Vipassana practice as giving her the psychological space to reform habits that 'disturb the balance of [the] mind.' But she did not feel able to transfer this disciplined equanimity to others while teaching *āsana*, until she discovered the little-known branch of Kashmir Yoga during a session on offer at Santosa. She says that Kashmir Yoga is 'not so much a tool as an idea', with a particular focus on experiencing the body during practice. From this point on, as an experienced post-lineage teacher, Veronika began to construct a hybrid method that combines the Ashtanga Yoga *āsana* repertoire, with tools for bodily self-awareness developed in Vipassana and Kashmir Yoga. Veronika is an accomplished teacher. Her taught and individual practice both consist of diagnostic movements to discern persistent and problematic neurological patterns, and movements designed to remove them. Each practitioner builds their

---

1 Unless otherwise stated, all citations in the case studies are by my respondents.

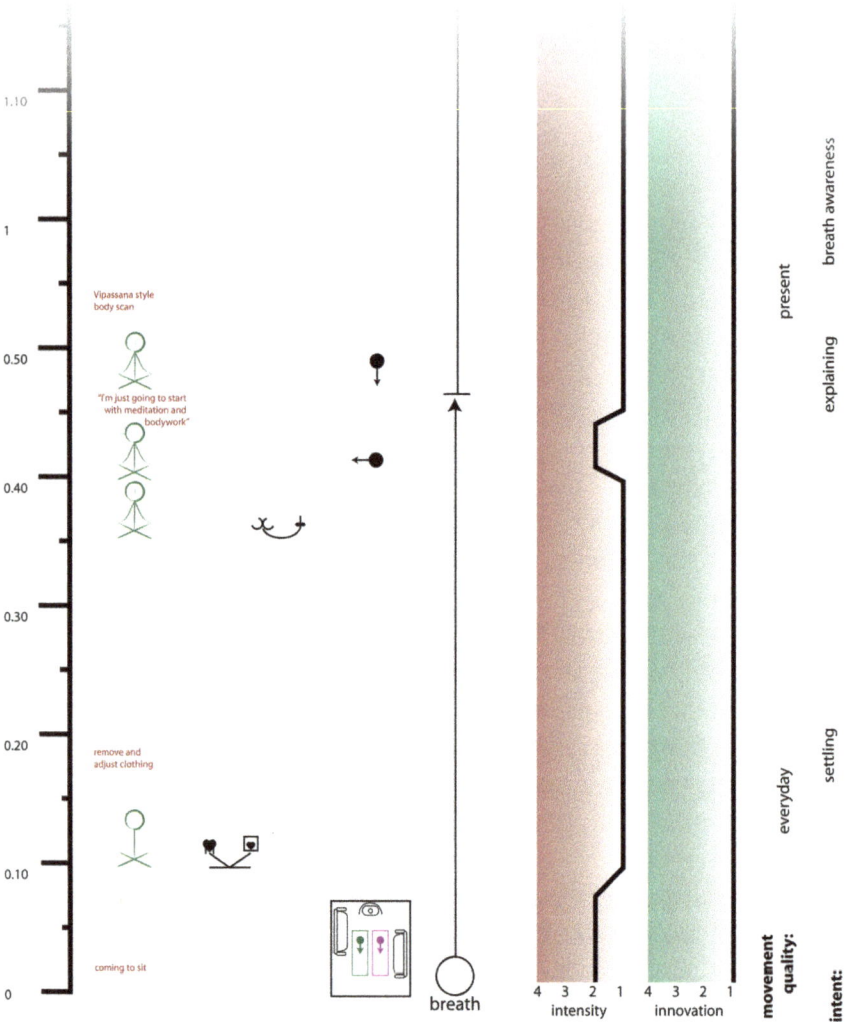

Figure 5.1
'The pristine body'

own practice, guided by the teacher to greater depths of internal awareness and discernment.

More recently still, Veronika and a colleague have further developed a lay understanding of infant neurology, exploring a therapeutic technique called the Rhythmic Movement Method, explained in Blomberg (2015). They were inspired by this to develop a practice that they call **Reflex**

Yoga, and a further specialism for autistic populations seen on their website (Zimbler 2017).

Living in Herefordshire, at home Veronika still teaches some Ashtanga Yoga, as it is much more popular in mainstream environments. But in contrast to those whom Veronika affectionately calls her 'Ashtanga hopping bunnies', the yoga she teaches at post-lineage community events is much slower and more mindful, characterised by a focus on incremental kinaesthetic transformation. Here, she labels such sessions as either Kashmir or Reflex Yoga, and uses the post-lineage network to promote and develop their work with neurodivergent populations.

Even though she lives close to a few like-minded teachers, Veronika also relishes the smaller yoga camps and gatherings for the profound sense of community they offer, and an ethical context that values frugality, compassion and ecology. She has been coming to Santosa and more recently Sundara, for many years. A humanist, Buddhist ontology precludes her from fully engaging with the community *kīrtan*s (devotional singing sessions). But she cherishes close personal bonds with many people here: 'It's the place where I fill myself up with all the energy I need to give back the yoga for the rest of the year.'

Through her practice, and her involvement in the *saṃgha* (spiritual community) of post-lineage yoga, Veronika seeks a way of being in the world that embraces a tension between three poles: acceptance of life's impermanent, imperfect, uncomfortable beauty; an incremental reclamation of a pristine original body; and faith in an eventual evolution to perfected awareness. Quoting Paul Fleischman, she says, 'You can never speak up too often for the love of all things, because "all things strive"' (Fleischman 2016).

LINEAGE AND AUTHORITY

At home, where we meet to practise together, Veronika does not have a separated space for yoga, and she rarely manages an uninterrupted daily practice: the demands of family pull on her. I can't use my yoga as an excuse or a reason not to be present [...] and just say, 'Sorry, I can't deal with you right now.'

For the sake of recording our co-practice session, her younger children are settled in the adjacent room, and Veronika manages a forty-minute practice, apart from one interruption 32 minutes in, when she goes to check on them before settling back into meditation.

The practice we explore together reflects Veronika's long history of multiple yoga and meditation influences. Our co-practice begins and ends with silent Vipassana meditation in the form of a breath awareness technique known as Anapana. Early in the practice, when Veronika has been consistently aware of the breath 'for a minute or so without interruption', she moves on to a systematic observation of the body in seated stillness. Consistent awareness of the somatic experience of the body gives way to practising equanimity to the sensations thus experienced. In the co-practice, this initial process takes around seven minutes in total.

Movement, when it comes, is steady, with few increases in intensity outside of periodic flowing sequences to keep the body warm. Veronika works from a well-established personal repertoire, including only what she already knows works for her. This includes a commonly adopted departure from the traditional Ashtanga Yoga *vinyāsa* (movement refrain) mentioned in Lutz (2015). We can see her in Figure 5.2, stepping forwards to kneeling rather than jumping through to sitting.

A number of movements during the co-practice are used to increase bodily sensation, such as opening and closing the palms. In this way, as she puts it 'you're actually constantly aware of the body in all its subtleties and all its gross sensations.'

These Vipassana and Kashmir Yoga techniques refine and intensify Veronika's somatic awareness so that the immediate needs of the body can be diagnosed internally. These are subsequently treated with movements from Reflex Yoga that she helped to develop, and sequences extracted from the set Ashtanga Yoga practice. Veronika contrasts the responsive somatic

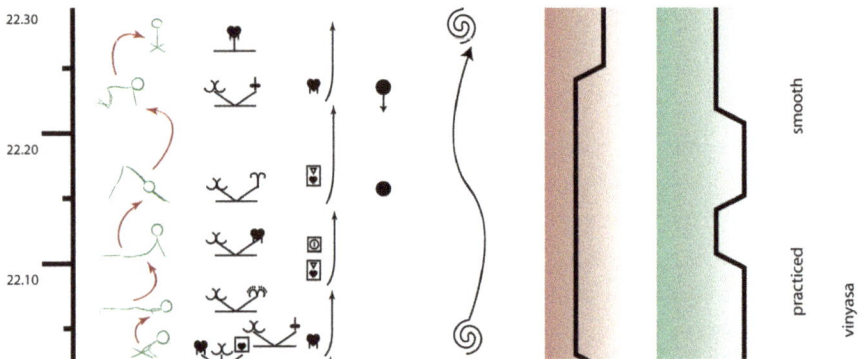

Figure 5.2
Adapting Ashtanga Yoga

awareness that is key to this way of practising, with those less-experienced practitioners whose practice is automatic rather than reflexive.

> You can tell by how they move. Yeah? If they move too fast, or too rhythmi-cally. Not even rhythmically. It's more habitually.

It takes many years to build both a personal repertoire of this kind, and the depth of bodily awareness needed to make choices about which ele-ments of practice to include each time a practitioner comes to their yoga mat. As a result, it is unclear whether the use of poses from the pre-set Ashtanga hip series to remedy the issues of the day is universally effective or a psycho-somatic effect entrained by Veronika's practice history and personal preferences.

INTENTIONS AND OUTCOMES

For Veronika's personal neurophysiology, a free, easeful breath is both the aim and result of her practice. Her chest often 'feels like a cage, [...] holding inside', preventing her from taking the breath that feels best for her. In an early forward bend, in Figure 5.3 she holds her head and checks the specific position of a particular vertebra that she feels 'dropping' if

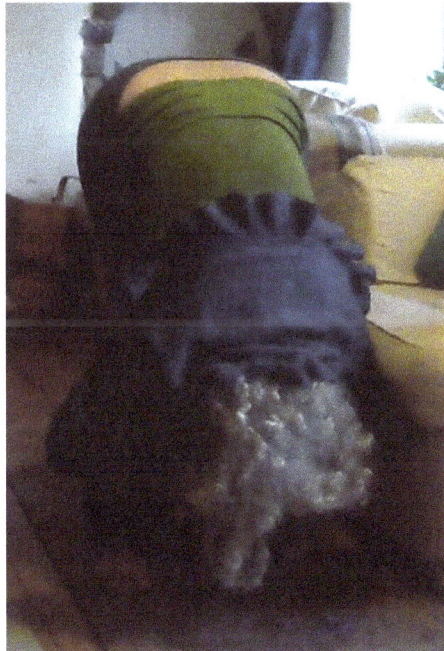

Figure 5.3
'Dropping' a vertebra

her breath is unencumbered. Elsewhere in the practice, frequent pauses allow her to match her experience against this primary objective of a free breath.

Twists and other cross-body movements in Figure 5.4 combine with a heightened awareness of the hands and breathing with the aim of

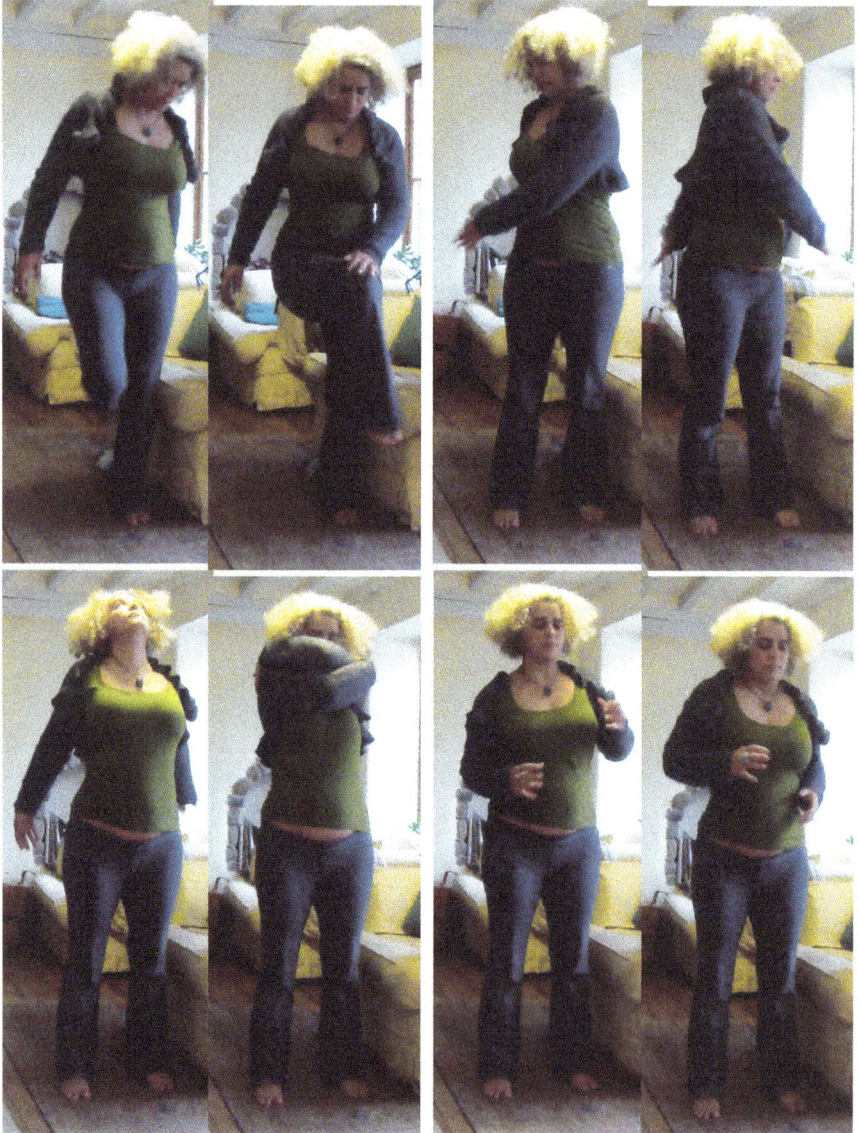

Figure 5.4
Clearing the 'Moro' reflex

awakening and clearing the relevant 'Moro' infant reflex pattern and lessening its recurrence.

The same pattern of movement and internal awareness is rehearsed in visualisation while performing more common *āsanas*. And Veronika knows that one particular bound twist, seen in Figure 5.5, gives her a better release of the breath than any other. After this peak twist has reset her breathing, she can explore taking that sense of ease into both movement and stillness.

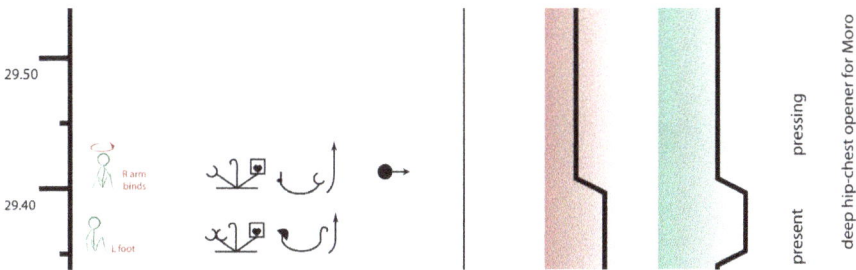

Figure 5.5
The peak twist

> And it's releasing even more, so I'm getting much, much deeper into that release, into that sense of teaching the body: you can be like this. [...] There's part of my neurology that knows that, yeah?

Veronika's practice balances between the equanimity of Vipassana, and the self-regulating protocols of her Reflex Yoga. It aims for sustainable maintenance rather than radical transformation. Incremental improvements bring novel experiences that feel familiar. She talks of evolving towards a bodily blueprint that was set before a history of common traumas set a less comfortable pattern in the body. This blueprint is both that of a familiar, younger body, and a more abstract ideal body requiring faith in its possible existence. 'Somewhere deep in there is [...] that deep knowledge, of that pristine body that you originally were.'

Her yoga practice allows her to intensify a somatic memory of feeling 'emotionally as well as physically open', and as a result, move more effectively in the world. As Vipassana resets her psychological processes, *āsana* resets her neurophysiology. As she understands it, we cannot control the events of our lives, but we can train for the most skilful responses. For

Veronika, evolving impermanence 'from breath to breath' is the only constant beyond that pristine blueprint.

Although she has had ecstatic experiences in yoga, she finds the concept of deity as implausible as a 'fairy tale'. For Veronika, humanity's unique gift is the capacity for self-awareness that makes conscious self-evolution possible. This transformation is the goal, but not the daily focus of her practice, which is in all forms a 'deliberate, determined act' to be present in equanimity. But the result can still be joyous, as seen in Figure 5.6.

> [It] doesn't teach you to be different. It teaches you to appreciate and have a love of all things, no matter what they are.

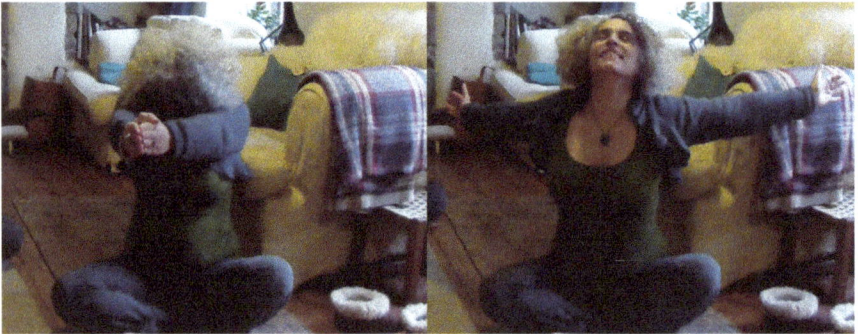

Figure 5.6
Enjoying a free breath

CASE STUDY 2
The 'microbial temple'

CHRISTOPHER

I was introduced to **Christopher** by Uma (Case study 3). There are significantly fewer men than women attending or teaching at most British yoga events, and he is one of the most well-known. Like Veronika in Case study 1, he first began as a student and teacher of Ashtanga Yoga, and his repertoire still holds many elements familiar to that system. After a similar journey to Veronika, through an even wider number of schools and lineages, he too settled on a personal specialism that moves beyond, but still honours, various lineages and teachers. In his case, this led to the development of what he named Engaged Yoga (Gladwell and Wender 2014). Engaged Yoga aims to be a fully holistic system for understanding and improving health and wellbeing, combining a range of philosophical, scientific and science-derived paradigms from Christopher's eclectic sources of inspiration. But although it aims to systematise, it does not make any claims to be the best or most correct form of yoga. Christopher has strong opinions on yoga, and indeed on life, relationships, and politics, but he holds the conviction that diversity and collaborative inspiration matter. Indeed, during my fieldwork he was exploring collaborative co-teaching with Uma, who has a very different practice indeed.

Christopher reads widely, and has written a number of books on yoga. He lives and works in Bristol, and teaches increasingly at low-impact retreat centres across Europe. He has not taught at Colourfest. At Sundara and Santosa he has been a charismatic presence and a high impact arrival, more likely to be engaged in intense debate than bonding over *sevā*. He is unselfconscious about his own practice, which is considered to be physically intensive. He practises publicly at events, and outside whenever he can, with as few barriers as possible between his body and the land, without the 'insulation' of mats or structures other people might consider practical or comfortable. For him, teaching at camps and retreat centres promotes a porousness of practice to place, and of the human to the wider-than human community of plants, animals and insects that form the local ecology.

Christopher – Friday 22nd April 2016, Bristol

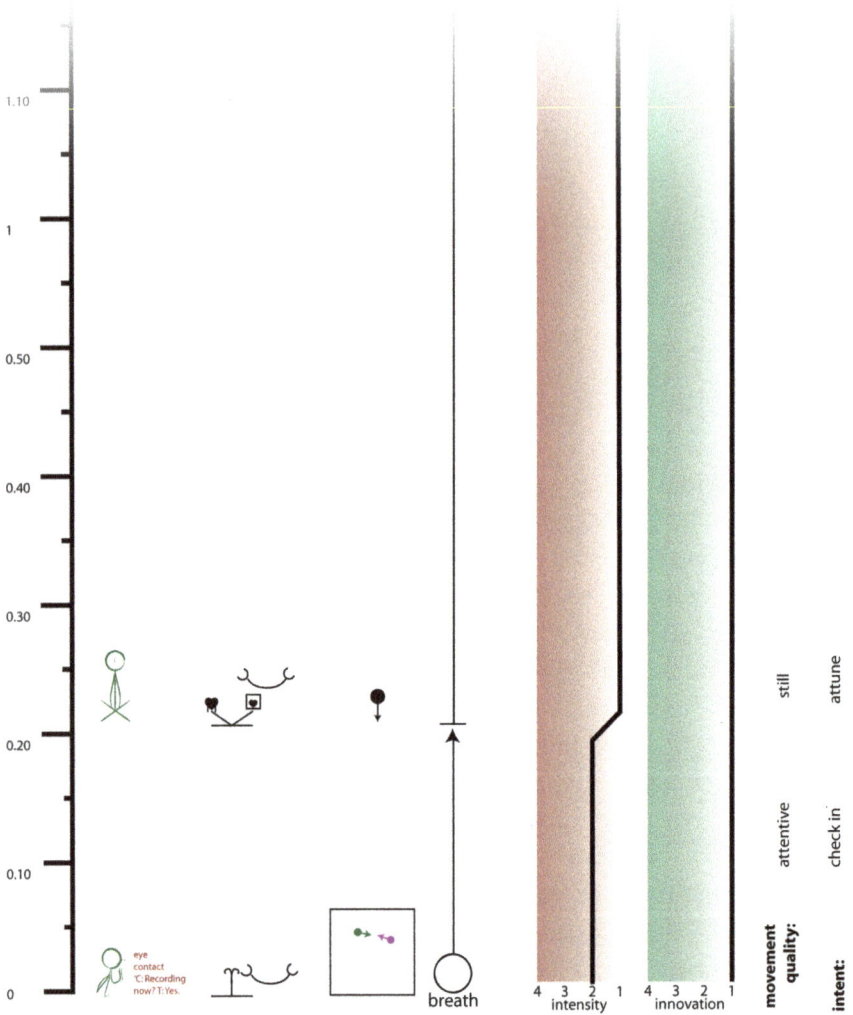

Figure 5.7
The 'microbial temple'

All this combines in Christopher's reputation for innovation, erudition and intensity, but it is the conscious and unconscious maintenance of his charismatic energy, and its effect within the subculture that most interested me about his practice.

His own experience of yoga began with a back injury:

I'd do visualisation practices [...]. And then moving in a way with my breath that felt right. [Then] somebody showed me a book with all these pictures of young people doing yoga and half the shapes I'd been making were in that book.

Later, one yoga school he studied with placed 'too much emphasis' on shoulder stands, another on long periods of sitting, both of which resulted in further injury. For Christopher however, injury is a near inevitable occasional result of moving through the world with an incomplete understanding of how the body responds. Christopher has his own definition of the 'guru principle', and how we as students can find the 'guru' as knowledge variously embodied in an external teacher, internal awareness, specific method or the universe. Yet, as he says, 'There's always that unknowingness which has to be engaged with in exploration, enquiry and dialogue.'

LINEAGE AND AUTHORITY

Outside in Christopher's suburban Bristol garden, our co-practice ecology includes rain, and the noise of traffic and construction. I am aware that Christopher has recently been in a traffic accident. We also discuss the effects of a microlight crash and the broken wrist he sustained coming off a bike eight weeks before. For Christopher, each of those impacts marks the porous body with the force of the world travelling to meet it. But responding effectively to injury for him is one route to increased resilience, as an opportunity for improved self-awareness.

Movement is like medicine, if you understand what you're doing [...]. We're pretty much a self-healing mechanism. Constantly seeking homeostasis and balance.

Yet a number of his early encounters with the universalised remedies of established yoga lineages left him with more physical issues rather than less. Christopher considers inept or inappropriate teaching to be a result of incomplete understanding of how life evolves and moves. The key to the practice, then, is listening to one's specific needs, as we learn to respond to the many stresses that come upon us as individuals, uniquely evolving in a robust world.

The practice he shares with me as a result is a contradiction of striving and gentleness. Cautious with his recent injuries, Christopher judges this day's *āsana* choices as accordingly exploratory and gentle, but by any other measure, this is a strong practice. Every section of practice is linked by a standard Ashtanga *vinyāsa*, with the addition of a pulsing bounce in *caturaṅga daṇḍāsana* (a low press up transitional position). Squats too are held with a pulsing bounce, working the muscles of shoulder and hip respectively. It is a practice that would be inaccessible to many practitioners, and unsustainable for others.

For Christopher, being sufficient to the needs of the world is enabled by regular efforts to train and test the self. His practice is precise, muscular, and functional, but so also esoteric in its quality of movement and its intentions. Even the stillness of meditation is a sprung tension of potential action in the world that gives the whole practice a sense of contained intensity. And yet Christopher's own experience of it is calm, gentle, even blissful.

From an initial attunement to the world, through each bowing reconnection to the earth and shift in gravity, in every testing exploration of balance, strength and mobility, his presence is as complete and sustained as the common and audible breath pattern that carries the practice known as *ujjāyī*. And if that practice may at times seem unforgiving, his quality of presence is one of care and intimacy. Whether this is effortless strength, or an internalisation of effort as normal, is ultimately unknowable to the researcher. Within historical and yoga debates, extreme, even supernatural powers are given as either an aim or side effect of practice (see Mallinson and Singleton 2017). In contemporary yoga such *siddhis* are often considered to be less important parts of historical source texts with uncertain ontological status (Wujastyk 2017). At the same time a hint of supernatural ability suggests a supernaturally dedicated practitioner. The charisma of many contemporary yoga teachers is to a large part based in the desirability of abilities such as hypermobility or acrobatic balancing that are almost supernatural and yet presented as mundane, and this is no different in the post-lineage subculture. Consciously or not, this is part of what Christopher is performing here.

According to Christopher, his practice restores function, increases understanding and resilience, and reclaims the union of self and world. His interpretation of ecological and socio-political disconnection is well practised. Missing from Christopher's narrative are the ways in which the limitations to personal power and possibility can persist beyond revealing the forces that create them. Although sequences of *āsanas* arise for him according to prior 'systems and preparation' and others relate to internal, energetic work, the shapes of Christopher's *āsana* and the refrain of *vinyāsa* are familiar from the Ashtanga practice repertoire, and its influence on modern postural yoga forms, as seen in practice guides such as Brown (2009). Even outside, his practice is largely linear, contained within the edges of the yoga mat he has left behind. Christopher is dismissive of what he calls the 'Hindu aerobics' led by teachers who are: 'just doing what they've been told.' But his own practice still shows its roots in what Alter has called 'muscular Hinduism', referring to postcolonial Hindu theological associations 'between muscles, morals and self discipline' (Alter 2006: 763) which greatly influenced the early modern development of yoga in India.

There are clear exceptions to this historical repertoire within Christopher's practice. Also included are functional engagements of the hips in squats, and the posterior muscle groups in active back bends. Fluid movement softens the edges of down dog and other variations familiar from the subculture's more 'feminine' practices. The graceful sideways lunge series in Figure 5.8 evokes a history with Chinese *qigong*. The influence of such 'functional movements', the practices labelled feminine, and martial arts are common within these practice networks, as Chapter 4 showed.

Christopher's unrelenting commitment to understanding the lived human condition, and his intimacy with the natural world, are foundational to his sense of self and his role in the world. This practice of deep somatic listening, is endless and evolving. Decades of experience have not

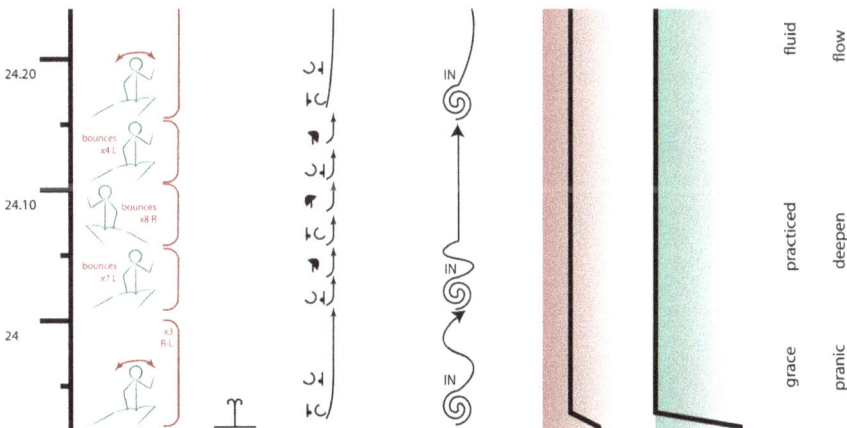

Figure 5.8
More fluid movement

dulled his drive to test the edges of the possible, to meet the world ever injured, ever healing, each and every day. As with Veronika, the practice incrementally evolves beyond lineage, keeping pace with the evolution of awareness.

> It's the movement in us for evolution and for change and for growth and for greater consciousness. It's something that just lives through us.

Christopher's focus is not on performance, however, but exploration of the moment to moment of lived, somatic experience. For him, each movement in the practice seeks an ever-shifting edge of possibility in action, within the arising boundary between internal and external world. For Christopher, this boundary exploration is the heart of the practice, and yet the boundary itself is also an illusion. As his own book describes it, much of the practice explores alignment to gravity, and strives to meet its force, as an expression of one's relationship to the ground of existence (Gladwell and Wender 2014). As a teacher, he sees much of his work as correcting a habit of 'over-extended' movement that is embedded in mainstream yoga teaching.

> That flow of tonnes of atmosphere through your body into the earth has to be channelled effectively.

The practice is also marked by frequent holds and gestures of binding the limbs around the body that explore, reinforce and then release more consciously drawn and evolving edges with the world, in the twists and folds seen in Figure 5.9.

This combination of intensity of effort, gentle presence, and explorations of gravity and edge are most evident in bound and held balances: the lotus variations of peacock and shoulderstand poses that come near the start and end of the practice. Before and after sit most of the less *āsana*-focused practices of breath, *bandha* (various body 'locks' or holding patterns) and meditation. Between them Christopher's dance with impact and strain, ease and connection, balances as if on a slackline, like the lotus peacock pose shown in Figure 5.10.

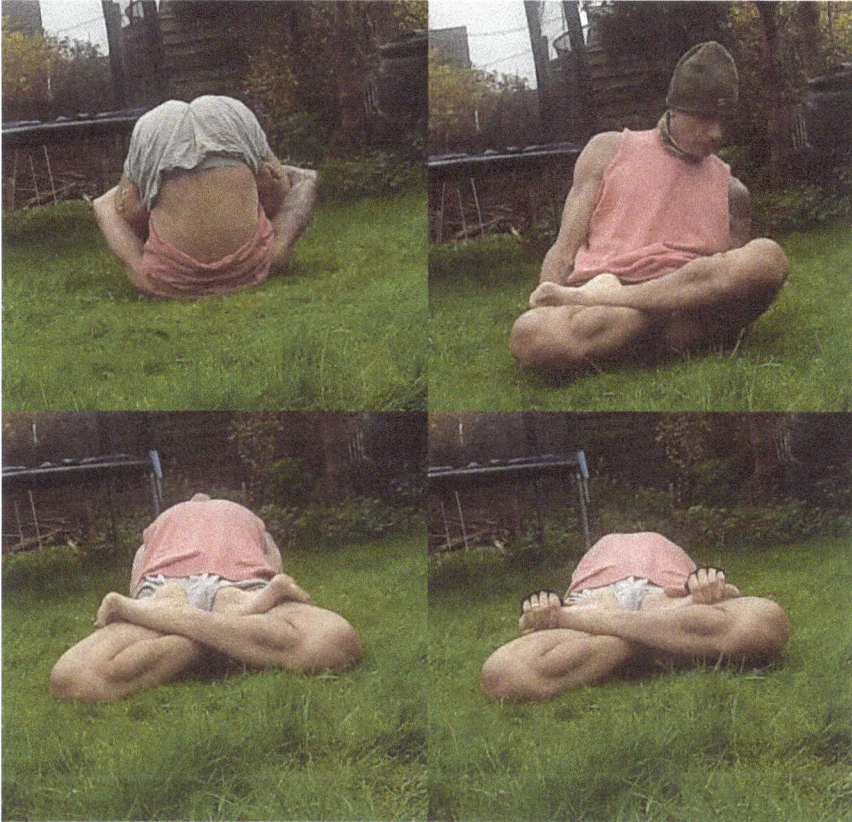

Figure 5.9
Holding and binding

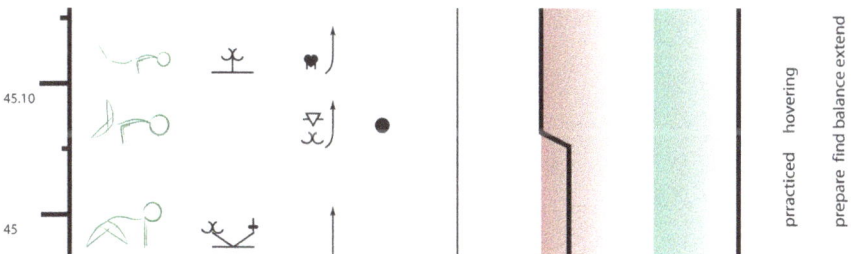

Figure 5.10
Balancing ease and strain

INTENTIONS AND OUTCOMES

Throughout the practice, Christopher is navigating trance states through pulsing movements, breath work, esoteric flows of energy and silently repeating *bīja mantra*s ('seed' or single syllable chants). Christopher wondered in the moment how to share these significant aspects without breaking his experiential flow. In the event, he trusts to the intimacy of mimesis and entrainment: the unconscious synchronisation between bodies. He speaks only to clarify two points of alignment, and share a momentary discovery in handstand. As he said to me afterwards: 'I could feel you feeling in. I could feel that relationship in fact as well.'

For Christopher, despite our resilient boundaries with a testing world, life is a presence that flows through all of us as sensation and receptivity. We are each a living temple temporarily holding space within the world for millions of sympathetic organisms.

> Most of the microbes that we host or that hold us together are really, really sweet ones. [...] If we feed them with the right stuff, they show us lots of love.

Thus, all practice is devotional to life itself, in a deliberate remembrance of porousness to the world. This remembrance is 'something that we need to practise daily because it's very easy to get lost in the unconsciousness of it all. In the nihilistic separate materialism.'

The illusion of separation is what he believes gives rise to the fortresses of rigid, artificial boundaries on the level of the corporation, religious institution or nation state just as much as within the individual person. Just as the canvas structures of camps and festivals enable a porousness of human to other than human presence, so at home in his garden, he is able to bring 'my own forehead the earth, to this holy, holy earth and [...] feeling the grass and the smell of the earth.'

Bound and yet finding freedom, he finds gratitude inevitable, reclaimed from the forces of ignorance and apathy, corporate 'beta-wave brain states' and other primitive, 'post-feudal nonsense'. As part of that porous unity of self-in-the-world, the presence of the researcher also affects the practice:

> The vortexes of peace and clarity that were there, it was just beautiful. [...] And I'm grateful because actually I think it was courtesy of this as well. [...] It's a really beautiful process. Thank you.

CASE STUDY 3
The dance of 'Śiva and Śakti'

UMA

As is true for many people, Uma was my own gatekeeper into the network. I first met her at one of her *yoganidrā* training courses. She is the founder of Santosa. Two other events (Sundara and Surya) have been founded by people who previously worked with her. A former Media Studies lecturer based between the alternative communities of Stroud and western Ireland, she maintains connections with teachers and scholars of yoga and Irish history alike, including friendships with a number of the Hatha Yoga Project team of scholars researching the pre-modern history of *āsana*.

She has been practising, and teaching for many years. When she was first a student, she would attend one studio teaching Sivananda Yoga, and another teaching Iyengar Yoga, and although she wasn't the only student to do this, she remembers both schools disapproving of this blending of sources. After training to teach Iyengar and Sivananda Yoga in turn, she moved on again, into the Satyananda Yoga community, where she met her husband, Nirlipta, who had been raised in the lineage. Indeed, she and Nirlipta were married not just by Swami Satyananda, but at his behest. She was later asked to leave a Satyananda Yoga teacher training, as she explains it, for asking awkward questions. During my fieldwork a major scandal broke within the Satyananda lineage that had a profound personal and professional impact on Uma and Nirlipta. By this point, Uma's work with pregnant and post-natal students had led to the creation of her own style of Womb Yoga, that aimed to correct the bias she saw within yoga teaching and philosophy, towards male bodies and experiences.

She has studied off and on for a number of years with Angela Farmer, another teacher exiled from lineage who is more influential than she is personally famous within European yoga culture, for, like Vanda Scaravelli, taking a perceived patriarchal practice of self-inquiry, and using it to explore the notion of the 'divine feminine' in movement practice. Angela Farmer, with her partner Victor van Kooten, were senior teachers of Iyengar Yoga, when Victor claims he was seriously hurt by Iyengar during

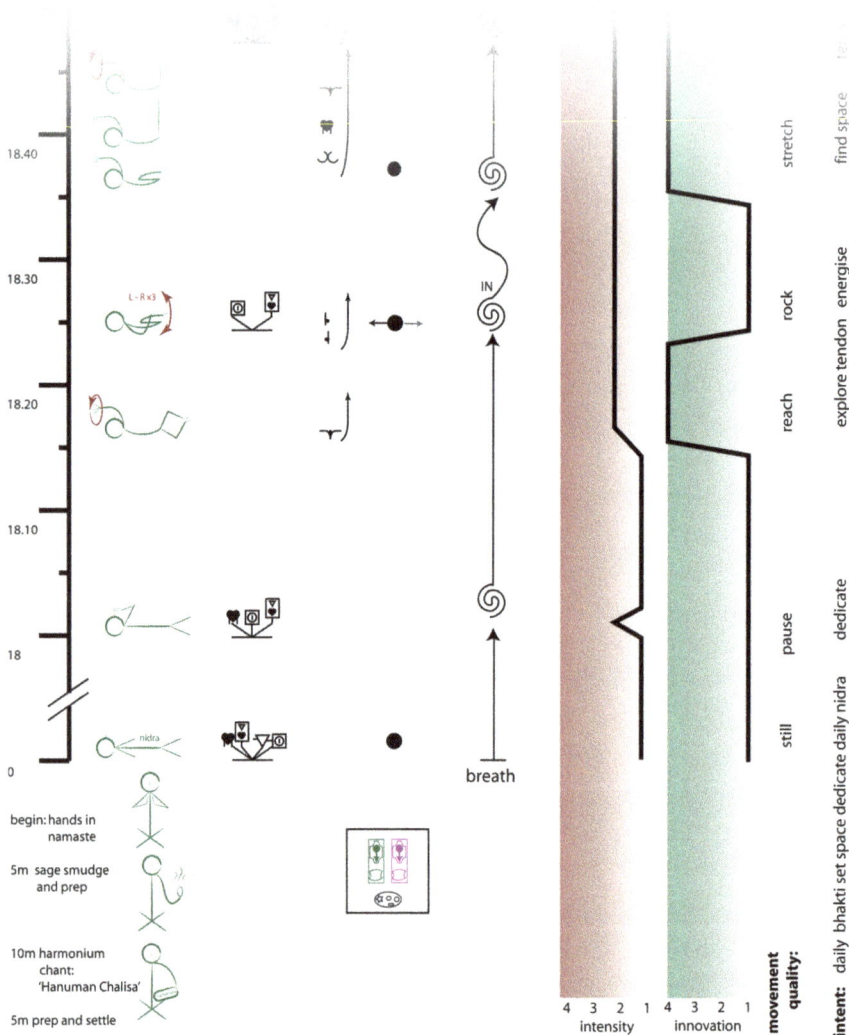

Figure 5.11
The dance of 'Śiva and Śakti'

a yoga practice, and it seems that both teachers were in some way black-listed or denigrated by the Iyengar organisation in return. This history is difficult to evidence, as the couple are quite private about the details, but they are part of the self-told origin story of this post-lineage subculture, and the story of radical female teachers who do not just move on from lineage but rebel against it, is a common one here.

Uma and Nirlipta also collaborated on developing a 'Total Yoga Nidra' training school for *yoganidrā* that seeks to combine the insights of multiple lineages in a way that recognises the benefits, limitations, and reasons for differences between them. In all this innovation, Uma and Nirlipta draw from a wide range of sources, benefiting from friendships not just with yoga teachers of numerous lineages, but with Sanskrit scholars, yoga historians, activists, psychologists and other medical professionals.

Uma teaches a highly recognisable practice. The unique circling refrain of hands and hips that form its core has spread through the post-lineage subculture from Uma's own Womb Yoga school (Dinsmore-Tuli 2013b). The quality of movement involved is entirely different from the linear and upright Mysore corpus, the precise internal oscillations of Angela Farmer seen in a film by Cummins (1997) and the drawings of van Kooten (1997), or the graceful flow of Scaravelli Inspired Yoga described in Scaravelli's own words (1991). It has more in common with the spontaneous ecstatic expressions of Sahaja Yoga (see Dharma 2017 for details) and Kripalu Yoga (see Kripalu Center for Yoga & Health 2017 for details) as described on their respective websites. Like them, this is a practice out on the wild edges of Tantric-inspired communion, but here, as I will show, it coalesces into a ritualised, repeated form, rather than endless innovation. As a result, it is much easier to teach to others.

This is also a profoundly emplaced practice, even as it is overlain with echoes of other places. Her practice is made in and reaffirms particular landscapes: Glastonbury, the Burren, the hills above Stroud. Uma thus also describes her practice as 'Celtic', in her co-written, inspirational manifesto for a Celtic School of Yoga (Dinsmore-Tuli and Harrison 2015). But her lifework to date is *Yoni Shakti* (Dinsmore-Tuli 2013b), a Tantric-inspired feminist guide to yoga that draws on little-known historical Tantric source materials.

As a response to the descriptions of *siddhi*s or yogic superpowers described in Patañjali's *Yogasūtra,* Uma has used the 'wisdom goddesses' of Śakta Tantra as inspiration for her categorisation of female superpowers (Dinsmore-Tuli 2013: 225). These female proto-*siddhi*s are based on natural, but not inevitable, female life events such as lactation and menopause. Uma considers them to be initiatory events with a capacity to provoke personal transformation. Uma is open about her role in this reimagining, while more commercially successful offerings of the 'divine feminine' are more likely to conflate the recently invented with long-standing traditions, as well as thoroughly essentialising gender and orientalising Hinduism (Maya 2015; Mantin 2004: 215).

Affinity groups from attendees of Uma and Nirlipta's courses, and readers of her books, form their overlapping peer networks. At Santosa Uma is a source of inspirational chaos and a referent for final authority. Supporting this is her conscious and community-building habit of celebrating and recognising the talents of others. This is as true when acknowledging her own teachers, such as Angela Farmer, as it is when honouring the volunteers that make her events possible. She has been immensely supportive of this research project. Like many of the dedicated teachers in post-lineage yoga, she is respected, but not famous, and once laughingly declared that taking part in the research made her 'feel more real as a result'.

LINEAGE AND AUTHORITY

On her way back from Ireland, where she has been planning a course on female sexuality and creativity, Uma asks if we can bring forward our scheduled time together, and the next morning I meet her in her converted garage studio in Stroud. The co-practice she shares is organic and expansive at nearly 2 hours long. It begins and ends in deep stillness.

Uma's practice dances with earth and air, fire and water: experiential categories of movement that she also associates with the masculine (fire) and feminine (water). As explained in the previous chapter, yoga for women's bodies is often explained within post-lineage yoga as a more nourishing practice. For Uma it is also responsive to the changing body and its ecology, and relies on an internal compass of authority.

Here these two nodes of masculine and feminine experience are in intimate relationship within the body of the individual practitioner, echoing and embodying the neo-Tantric divine dance of Śiva and Śakti, and also the love of Sītā and Ram in the Ramayana. Uma makes a concrete connection between the latter myth and her own marriage, in discussing the complicated history of their involvement with the Satyananda Yoga lineage.

> [My husband and I] were [Satyananda's] *mūrtis*. [...] He worshipped Sītā and Ram. [...] and even then, there was something in my little feminist defended cunt place that was like: there was something weird [happening].

Pavanamuktāsana (joint mobilisation) movements are derived originally from Satyananda Yoga (for a definitive practice guide to Satyananda Yoga, see Saraswati 2013). In this co-practice, they are given a 'feminine, soft' edge, inspired by the teachings of Angela Farmer. These are practices for what Uma 'always felt were vulnerable female bodies' until she 'realised that everybody is vulnerable'. As Uma explains it, long term individual practice enables the self-knowledge needed for female practitioners to resist the authoritarian and universalising tendencies of masculine yoga systems. Yet Uma herself is proof that a similar depth of individual practice is also what confers charismatic authority on to all teachers, regardless of gender.

Uma frequently describes the relationships between male and female practitioners and yoga teachers in terms of intimacy, power and danger. Charismatic, masculine teaching includes 'money and sex and bodies and intimacy', while teachers such as Angela Farmer create a less 'virile', more consciously post-lineage space of re-enchantment in a form of intimacy with one's ecology and every part of the physical self.

It is in this dance between universalising masculine authority and the feminine invitation to self-intimacy that Uma sees her practice, and post-lineage yoga, evolving. An overtly feminist reworking of the practice begins when you take the practice 'into the laboratory of your own self'. This process of reclaiming however holds the risk of disempowerment, when patriarchal, corrective gazes over largely female bodies are legitimised within wider yoga culture.

For Uma, the visceral, female self is the centre of her practice, explored through wriggling, spontaneous movements such as those in Figure 5.12. For her, this visceral female self will on occasion respond instinctively to the threat of patriarchal authority with spontaneous purification. Arriving at one ashram, Uma suddenly started:

> Unstoppable *kuṃjal* [an emetic purification practice] until I couldn't vomit anymore [...] and I said 'You have to take me out of this place'.

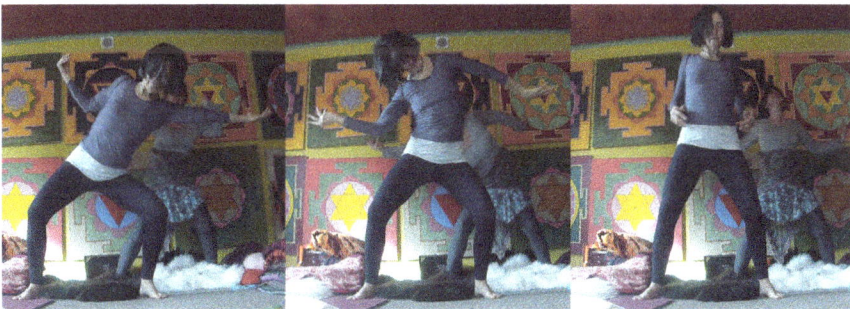

Figure 5.12
Exploring the visceral, female self

Other practices from patriarchal systems, such as Satyananda's Yoga Nidra and *pavanamuktāsana* might be reformed through individual practice, to serve more liberatory, inclusive aims. As she asks:

> [If] I'm tied up in knots with a belt holding me around, [...] why is that okay? [...] I've been held in a space of intimacy that's allowed for that to happen because I've taken it away and practised it.

INTENTIONS AND OUTCOMES

Throughout the co-practice, Uma's eyes mostly stay closed, yet like Christopher (Case study 2) she repeatedly renegotiates boundaries: wrapping and removing blankets, and adjusting how her body meets the ground. Rocking refrains of movement flow almost always in time with a conscious breath, exploring a position in a series of waves, like a rising and falling tide. Movement is accompanied by sighs and shakes and groans.

Uma practises in both the search for and the appreciation of what she defines as a sense of 'space opening up in the body'. Each exploratory movement is repeated with micro-adjustments in joint position that test the limits of movement as if refining its target. Each ends with shaking out a body part, expelling somatic tension before returning to an evolving refrain of circling hips and elegant *mudrā*s shown in Figure 5.13. Some of the most intense moments of the co-practice are also those of high innovation: a sensuous search for the sensation of release through effort.

Within the co-practice are shapes that reflect Uma's more conventional yoga history of Sivananda, Iyengar and Satyananda Yoga. These include supine stretches and seated hip variations. Uma also explores more precise shapes for her tendonitis, learned in recent practice with Christopher.

The circling refrain of hands and hips that form the core of the practice, and the heart of her own Womb Yoga style, lends an energetic, bent-elbowed, squatting, and wriggling pulsation to the rest of this co-practice.

Uma describes the intent for the co-practice as a combination of connecting the feet to the earth, honouring the womb as she is late bleeding, and rehabilitation for chronic tendonitis on her left (dominant) side, including moments of self-massage seen in Figure 5.14.

Despite the somatic sensuality of the practice, when asked, Uma says her practice is about 'maintaining a degree of flexibility, strength and mobility that helps me get on with my life without having to think about my body. [...] I want to just enjoy being in it.'

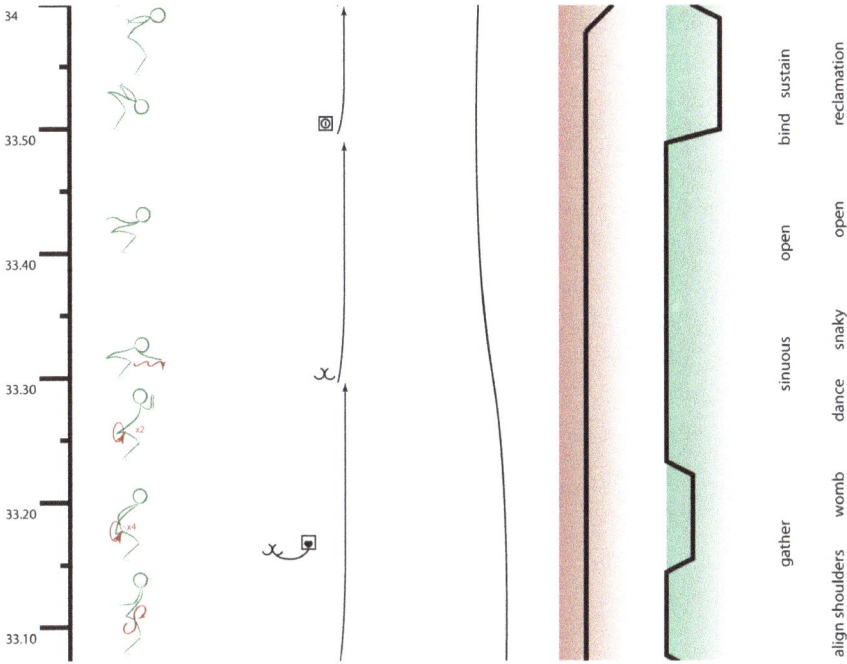

Figure 5.13
Intensity and innovation

Each sensory engagement with immediate ecology is a pulsation: reaching out and drawing back in to process sensory input. Uma associates 'thinking about the body' with discomfort, and freedom from pain with sensual delight and a lack of rational involvement with bodily demands. She balances 'what feels good' in the practice with her experiential knowledge of what feels beneficial in the long term, but her reward is immediate and joyous. 'I get off on it. [...] It's like making love with yourself.'

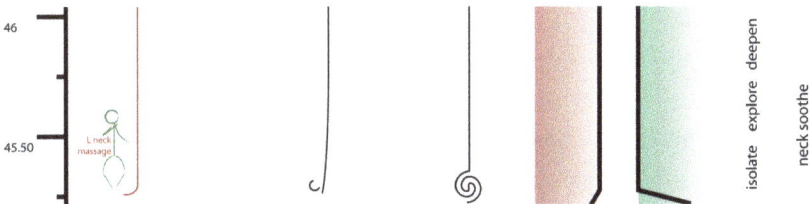

Figure 5.14
Self-massage

Uma explains the co-practice as a journey through five porous elemental categories of earth, water, fire, air and aether. The *āsana* portion begins lying supine, preceded and literally grounded in a self-guided *yoganidrā* accompanied by the recorded sounds of a river in the Burren, Ireland. Her connection to land and earth, remembered through the feet in standing, is transformed through water, which she explores as flowing, lubricating movements of pulsating waves in the body. Fire is invoked in more internal pumping motions that accompany the increase of intensity. Here, variations of *uḍḍīyana bandha* and *mūlabandha* like the one seen in Figures 5.15 and 5.16, draw up the diaphragms of the abdomen but are integrated into movement rather than more traditionally performed in static shapes. They are also modified to release down as well as rise up.

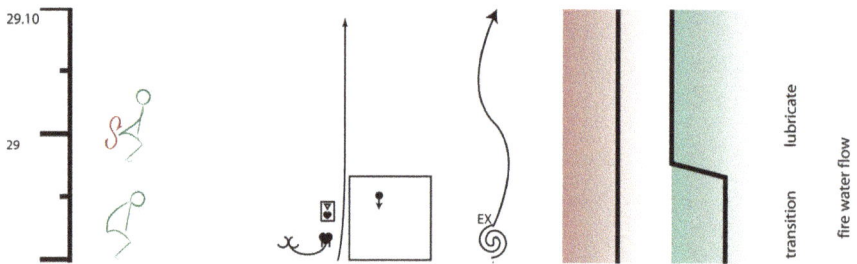

Figure 5.15
Adapting bandhas

Uma claims to use fire to pump the energy of the earth from the feet, having made it fluid, and then expands it into airy breath, embodied in expansive arm gestures made precise by the illumination of mindfulness. The practice energetics are refined finally into aether, ending 'with sound and *mantra* and silence.'

That returns the practice to stillness, and devotion. Throughout, Uma's hands frequently come to the heart or the forehead in a universal gesture of prayer, and the practice settles with a final meditation with a Tibetan *trenwa* (*mālā* or rosary). She performs two silent rounds of *mantras*, followed by a seated *nyāsa*: an internal practice inscribing the devotional body from within with imagined symbols.

Uma links this devotion to borrowed lineage, through friends in the Tibetan Aroter and Hindu Babaji communities. Embodied in the 'authentic

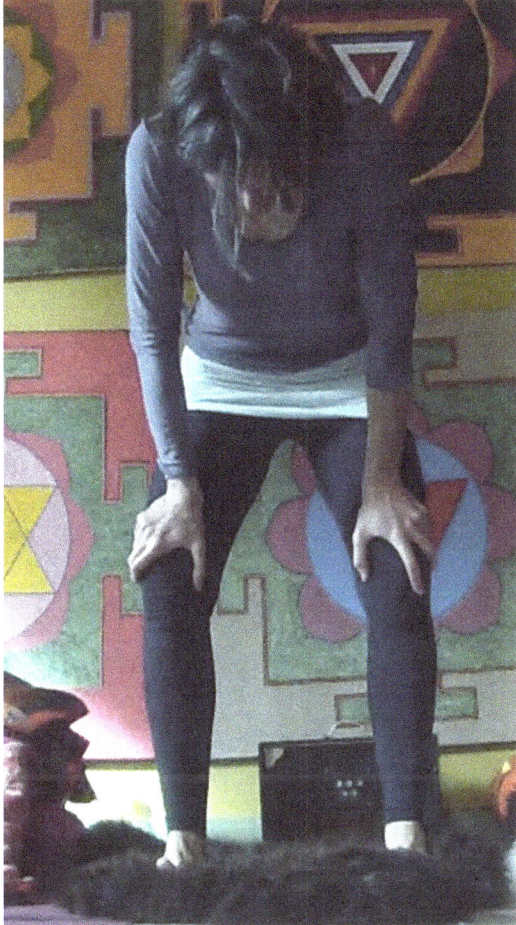

Figure 5.16
Adapting bandhas

and old' gifts of *mūrti*s, rosaries and temple bells, she talks about this part of the practice more as a link to community than guru, and land rather than deity. For her they are a collection that mixes symbols of her relationships within a gift economy, with found natural treasures.

CASE STUDY 4

'Part of you and part of nature and everything'

SIVANI MATA

Sivani Mata's journey to post-lineage yoga began, like many, with Ashtanga Yoga. She left this behind in search of a practice that was less prescriptive, and more adaptable to her own biological rhythms, and trained with Uma (Case study 3). She now travels to teach on both Total Yoga Nidra and Womb Yoga workshops and courses, but she also leads her own retreats, and travels widely as a *bhakti* musician, leading *kīrtan* on her own events and those of others. This brings her into collaboration with even more teachers, and a wide range of schools and influences. I met Sivani Mata through Uma, but spent most time getting to know her through camping side by side at Colourfest. As a result of her eclectic personal journey, Sivani Mata is involved in a number of key smaller affinity groups within the subculture. She is an established feature of both Colourfest and Santosa schedules. Her own music is inspired by relatively obscure *bhakti* poets such as the eleventh-century Lalla Ded.

Alongside this journey of personal exploration, for many years, Sivani Mata has also identified as part of the Babaji lineage community, mentioned previously, one of numerous Hindu saints known as Babaji whose hagiography can be found at Samaj (2017). She is one of the Babaji Temple Singers who lead *kīrtan*, ritual and events throughout the year. But in the absence of the physical presence of the (dead or ascended) guru, she adapts her personal and taught practice as inspiration and experience dictate. The heart of Sivani Mata's practice as seen in the next chapter, is a *pūjā* form that is practised at all three events profiled in this book, and more besides. With this form Sivani Mata blends Womb Yoga practices, *yoganidrā*, and her own *bhakti* songs. She is also trained to teach Shakti Dance, described earlier in this chapter. Shakti Dance is itself a blend of Kundalini Yoga with elements from ecstatic dance and other traditions, and thus, Sivani Mata chooses elements of practice day by day, from a range of sources that form her personal history of practice, to fit around her regular *pūjā* structure in ways that would contradict the direct teachings of most *bhakti* lineages.

Sivani Mata – Thursday 21st April 2016, London

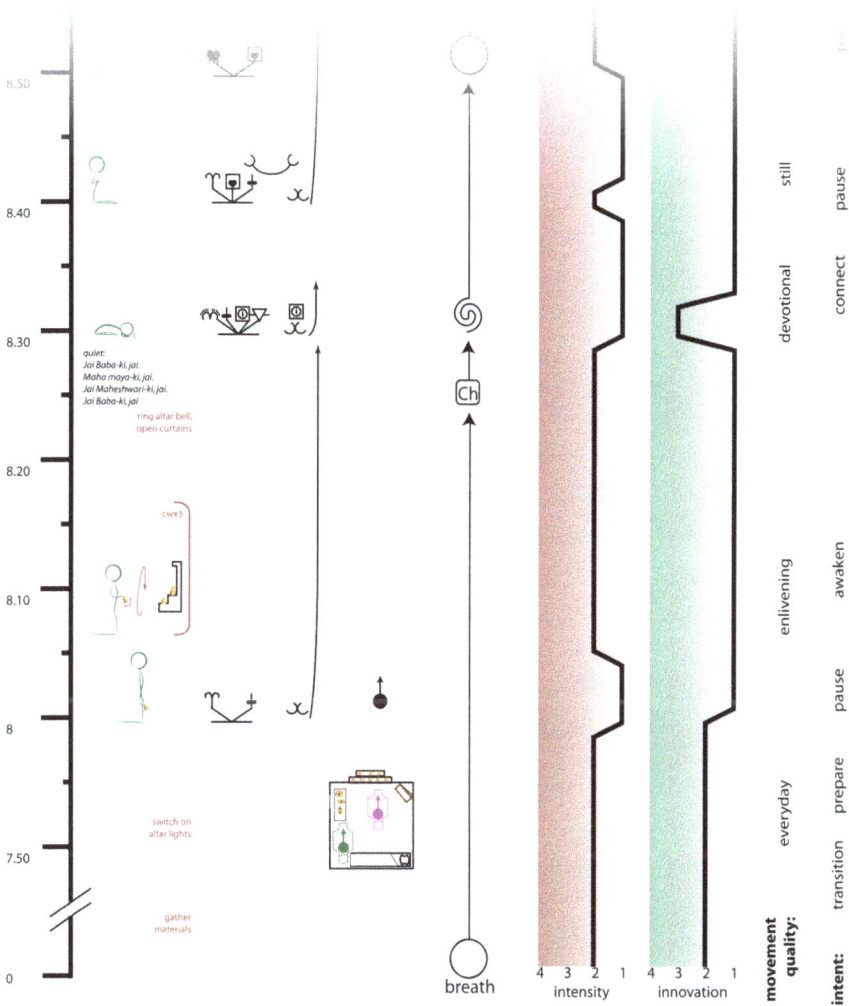

Figure 5.17
'Part of you and part of nature and everything'

Her practice is most interesting because of how she blurs the boundary between *bhaktiyoga* and *āsana*, or yoga, music and dance. Prior to yoga, her countercultural roots lie in underground rave culture. The various events she teaches and performs at maintain her connections to all of these and more.

> I entered the jasmine garden
> where Śiva and Śakti were making love.
> I dissolved into them
> I dissolved into them.
>   (Francis 2017, based on a poem by Lalla Ded)

LINEAGE AND AUTHORITY

In Sivani Mata's small bedroom in the London home she shares with her mother, we gather as she puts together her supplies, and begin a co-practice that is a spacious 90 minutes long, including her most intimate daily devotions.

Sivani Mata adapts some aspects of the set *pūjā* of her Babaji lineage in order to better reflect what she considers to be their deeper purpose. Other aspects of ritual are retained, but only after exploring their effects. Like Uma, she also adopts a more radically feminist reclaiming of some traditional taboos. She refrains from full *pūjās* during her monthly bleed not because it is impure, but because 'I don't need this full-on practice. I'm already making offerings. *Yoni puṣpam.* I'm offering flowers everywhere. It's perfect!'[2]

Her repetition of daily ritual actions therefore is practised rather than automatic, with an economy of movement that leaves space for innovation and attentive lived experience. Each *mūrti* has their own pattern of anointing. Each day a different perfumed oil and *mālā* is used.

Movement and song are the most spontaneous sections of the practice. Movement begins, as in Figure 5.18, with a simple rocking of the spine. This follows the breath, then evolves smoothly into more expressive, pulsing *āsanas*. Each movement has a dynamic, organically emerging and consistent form. These echo many of the Womb Yoga shapes, but stay within a gentler rhythm than Uma's co-practice. Each *āsana* is performed with the skilled application of appropriate force that can be interpreted as grace. Movement flows out of the breath as if inherent to bodily structure.

Breath is the origin point for movement, which becomes a dance of offering, which becomes song in turn, in the long and hypnotic, repeating chants that are her hallmark as a musician. Most of those songs are in Sanskrit. This is a language she reserves for connecting 'with creation on a

---

2 One term for menstruation in yogic discourse, taken from the Sanskrit, is *yoni puṣpam*, translated as 'flowers from the source'.

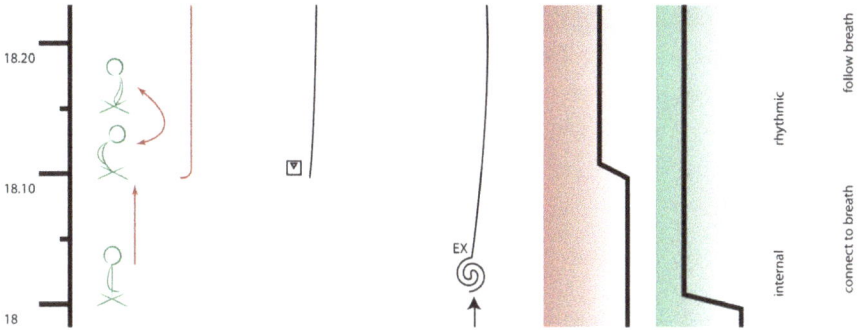

Figure 5.18
From breath to movement

higher level'. Like the group practices discussed in the previous chapter, all of them rise steadily out of, and return to stillness, just as the *āsana* practice flows out of and returns to seated and largely still breathing practices.

The heart of Sivani Mata's practice is her *pūjā* to an altar of mostly, but not entirely Hindu *mūrtis*. Unlike the *pūjā*s that take place at post-lineage events, led by ritualists of the Babaji, Amma or Integral lineages, however, the elaborate and repeated gestures of surrender and rituals of washing, feeding and anointing are here part of individual rather than communal acts of devotion. The overall structure diverges in significant aspects from the lineage form, not least in including *āsana* at all, and each day varies as to how much time is spent on each element.

> It is traditional to do *nāḍī śodhana* at that point and then just move straight into washing. So that feels like the natural pause [for movement].

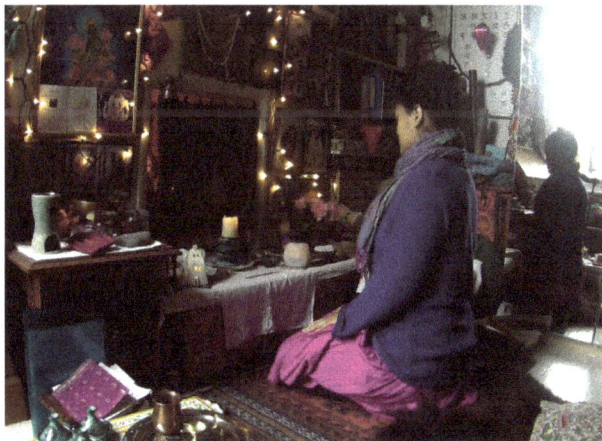

Figure 5.19
A space filled
with ritual objects

For Sivani Mata, the rhythm of washing and anointing itself is 'like a very intimate moving meditation'. Her ritualised movements interact with the space, involving more than the usual yoga mat and cushion or sheepskin. In fact, as seen in Figure 5.19, above, a yoga mat would not fit in this place, crowded with ritual paraphernalia and instruments.

INTENTIONS AND OUTCOMES

Through the *pūjā* Sivani Mata expresses a fluid permeability between *mūrti*, deity and self. The animating practice that breathes ongoing life into the *mūrti*, breathes life again into a remembered perfection of the self.

> Some people really feel like the *mūrti* is the being. On one level, I feel that, but [also] part of you and part of nature and everything.

Following ritual cleansing, offerings are made to the *mūrtis* and then imbibed by the bodily self, and smoke, light and song are washed over the altar, the self and the space. These forms of multiple cleansing and multiple nourishment intensify the porousness of identity and strength of identification of self to deity and place. The entire co-practice is held by the tiny room to which she retreats to sleep and worship, in the heart of her home. Within the room's larger altar is an inner hearth, protected by a curtain behind which the chosen *mūrtis* of the day will eat. In Sivani Mata's narrative, layers of self and other together multiply and are each intimately enclosed in a nurturing ecology that provides a sense of sanctuary. We discuss the intimacy of filming in the practice space, which she describes as 'a bit like taking a picture of my *yoni* [vulva]!'

Despite these layers of separation, this is more of an oasis than a monastic cell, a garden tumbling over the edges of its urban plot. The layers of internalisation create a deliberate space at their heart for the most delicate processes of personal healing. Within, the oasis of practice can function to reframe the mundane issues of the self through self-divinisation.

> I'm kind of trying to get out my shell a bit again. I'm in a quite deep healing process and I've been kind of allowing that to take over my life a bit.

The intimate and enclosed relationship between deity, *mūrti* and self, is a negotiation between the mundane and the divine in the same body. It is expressed in narratives of burying and unearthing that which seems ugly and beautiful about the self, in the surfaces and depths that form identity. Sivani Mata has been healing from a long-held pattern of burying grief that she sees manifest as eczema on the surface of her skin.

Sivani Mata aims to train the self with nourishment rather than discipline. Both self-nourishment and offerings to deity arise from the same reclamation of abundant delight. For her, the path of *bhakti* is:

> To delight in one's true nature and [...] 'Oh, what a joy it is to be in this body and to be in this world and to notice the beauty and love in the world.'

This sense of delight is a deeper truth she can reconcile with experiences of grief and disease. Delight at being 'at one with the earth and the dirt [...] as well as the purity and everything that is up' is her eventual aim, with her feet on the bare earth. Sivani Mata balances above the two fallen states of mundane self-pity and denial of the lived experience. Deities such as the ones chosen in this co-practice that express abundant beauty, humble rootedness and these contradictions of 'shadow' and 'light' are particularly loved.

Sivani Mata talks less of her relationship to the guru, and more of the archetype of Babaji as both worldly and divine. For her, the tiny *mūrtis* of his sandals being washed are the perfect embodiment of the everyday meeting points between human and divine, earth and sky. Our rightful state is between what she calls the 'love making' of earth and sky, in which, experiences of the sacred can spill over into a more delighted experience of everyday lived experience.

Despite the multiply protected practice space, and numerous ritual actions that involve purification by water, light, or smoke, Sivani Mata dislikes yoga traditions and teachers that are obsessive about separating the sacred from the mundane. This is particularly the case for those that consider female bodily processes to be unclean, or seek to distance themselves from the influence of rave culture on British yoga. Sivani Mata draws a connection between her accidental experiences of trance in a rave setting and her practice now, and the event she attends most assiduously is that with the most overt rave influences: Colourfest. She says: 'I mean, Shpongle and Prem Joshua let me find *kīrtan*.'[3]

---

3 Respectively, Shpongle and Prem Joshua are a psychedelic trance duo and a world music act, both producing music with Hindu devotional elements.

For Sivani Mata *bhakti* denies neither other possible routes to devotion, nor the mundane world. An hour of ritual cleansing reclaims the pre-existent perfection of self, *mūrti*, world and deity. Offerings of fruit and light and voice express a remembrance of abundance. Movement (as in Figures 5.20 and 5.21) and song are an artist's reclamation of holistic beauty. Sivani Mata's practice is deliberately grounded, but graceful rather than visceral.

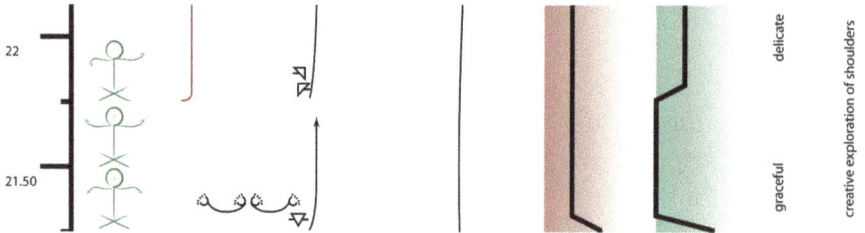

Figure 5.20
Grace in movement

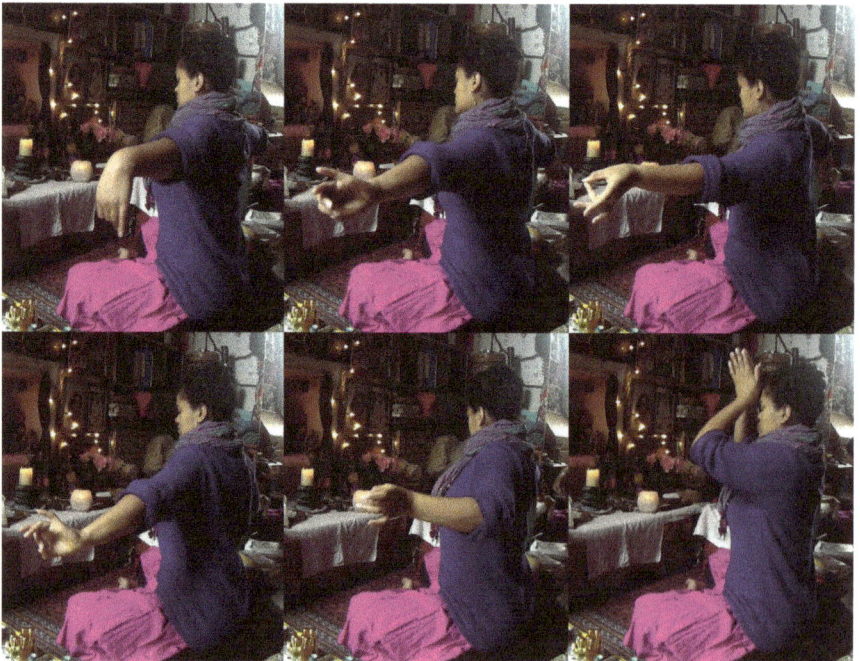

Figure 5.21
Grace in movement

CASE STUDY 5

'Building nerves of steel' with building blocks of practice

TANYA

Tanya's yoga history began by practising with a local Hatha Yoga teacher. Later, a trip to India was inspired by a dream revelation:

> I [...] was given two words. One was Navaratri and one was Babaji.

While in India for the Navaratri celebrations at the Babaji ashram, she and her husband were then inspired to travel to Mysore and train as Ashtanga Yoga teachers. The *āsana* sequences and 'strong connection[s]' that they learned and formed there sustained Tanya's teaching and practice for many years. Alongside this, she made connections to, and continues to spend time with the Babaji and also Osho lineage communities, but committed exclusively to neither these, nor to the Ashtanga Yoga community. As part of her own journey into parenthood, she trained in Pregnancy Yoga with Uma (Case study 3), and as a result, discovered this post-lineage community.

It was at Santosa that Tanya first encountered Kundalini Yoga: 'I knew that that was the yoga for me in that moment.' She trained to teach Kundalini Yoga, and now when she teaches, mostly teaches from that repertoire, adding in elements of Hatha Yoga and Ashtanga Yoga and more, whenever she feels it useful. But the teachers she invites to the gathering she runs with John, her husband, teach a wide range of more and less well-known forms, and show evidence of an eclectic range of sources.

Tanya's individual practice, her public image and her teaching are closely related. The *method* of Kundalini Yoga is much more foundational to Tanya's practice than the ongoing influence of any specific teachers who have taught it. But Tanya does defer to the authority or at least experience of wiser beings who have walked the human journey before us. And the authority of the guru archetype for her is not restrained to lineage, nor to the ideal of rare beings with profound yogic knowledge. Anyone in the human family can be a teacher for her, and thus the act of coming

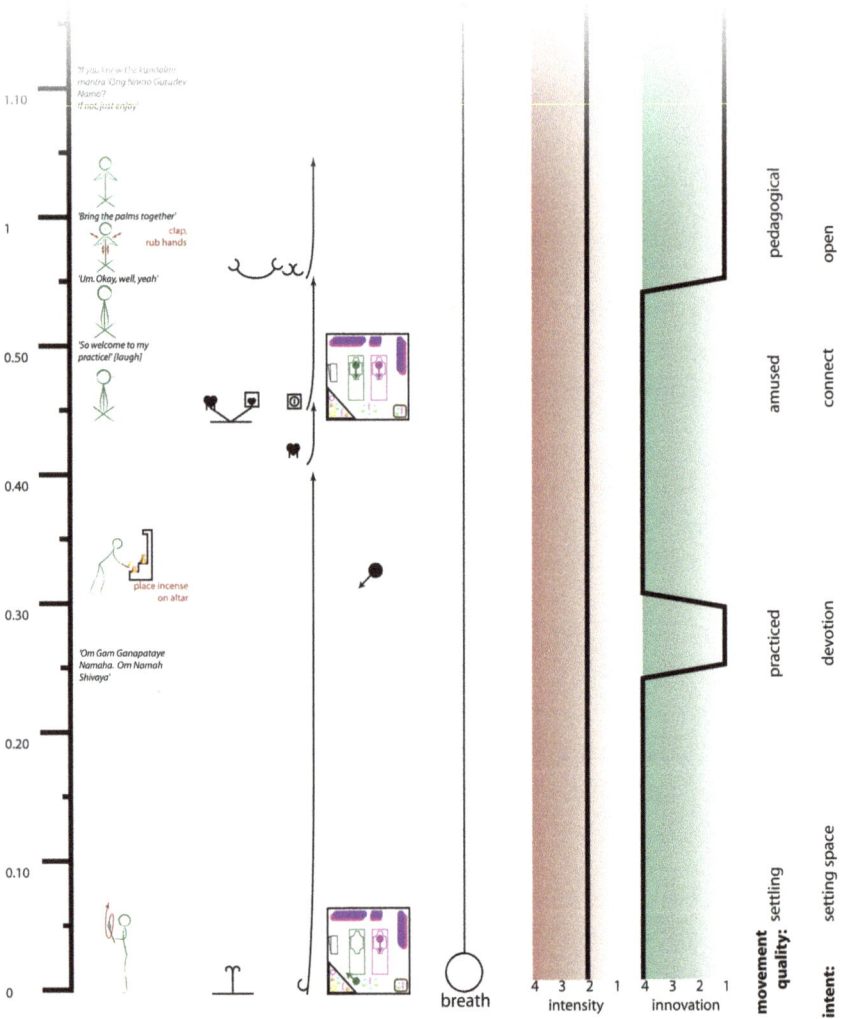

Figure 5.22
'Building nerves of steel'

together at these events enables more of those inspirational encounters to happen. Tanya's own first inspiration was her grandmother.

> There was [...] this absolute grace that I never saw in anybody else. [...] I think it was through her that I really knew that some people were different to others.

Unusually among these case studies, Tanya has named no style of yoga, and written no books. Yet like Uma, she is one of the most well-connected figures in the subculture. As well as organising Sundara, and working at Colourfest, John and Tanya also run a chai tea stall at other post-lineage events, often for charity, including the Beltane Bhakti Gathering mentioned previously. For both of them the running of events is, as explained previously, a long-held habit.

LINEAGE AND AUTHORITY

We settle into Tanya's tiny yoga room where a corner altar overflows with *mūrtis*, crystals, incense and flowers. Behind us is a stack of bolsters and blankets for teaching yoga. Our co-practice begins with *mantras* and contemplation, during which the aim and form of the session intuitively arise for Tanya. This is followed by a few basic stretches like the ones in Figure 5.23, and the Kundalini Yoga practices of *ṣaṭkriyā*, and the first of many variations of the pumping breath of fire, instructions and context for both of which can be found on the 3HO website (Bhajan 2008b). Breath of fire is a forceful breathing practice common in Kundalini Yoga, used to create heat and energy in the body, and a common feature of various sessions at the event she organises, Sundara.

After a more generic Hatha Yoga sun salutation, the main body of the co-practice is a much more complex Kundalini Yoga sequence of combined breath, movement and *mantra* designed to activate the pituitary gland. Following this, a short *śavāsana* (supine rest) with crystals laid on the body provides another intuited answer for the following part of the

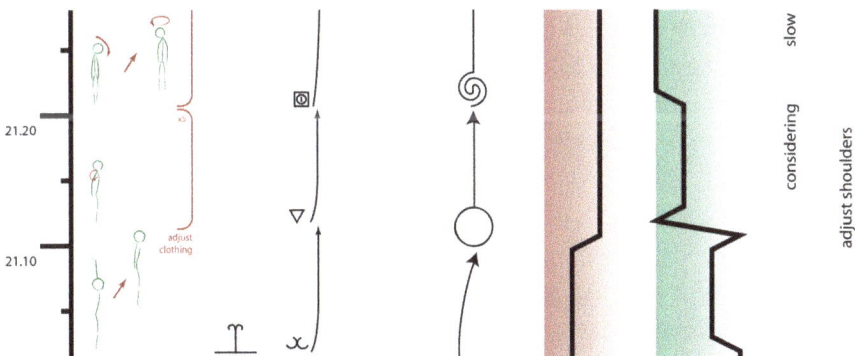

Figure 5.23
Starting stretches

practice: a Kundalini Yoga meditation 'for ending habituation patterns' (Bhajan 2008a), and another to 'rebuild the identity' that includes a complex ***prāṇāyāma*** (breath practice) involving suspending the breath for set periods (Bhajan 2017). The final part of the session is a *bhakti* practice also influenced by the Babaji lineage: chanting, stillness, and prayers to close.

Throughout, Tanya's relationship to the practice is steady and controlled. Shapes are often held for a specific length of time, according to pre-set instructions, to serve a particular internal energetic effect. Like my other case studies, Tanya combines traditions without adherence to any single teacher. She describes herself as a follower of 'the path of love and service'.

> It really is on a day-to-day basis. If I wake up tomorrow morning and I'm not feeling Kundalini Yoga, I don't do Kundalini Yoga.

Movements are drawn from a range of sources, and some are spontaneous or adapted. But when performing the Kundalini Yoga sequences Tanya adheres closely to orthopraxy. She offers the possibility of using 'the *Vedas* or the ancient Sanskrit scriptures' to put one's own *kriyās* (cleansing practices) together. But in her experience repeated practice leads to a deeper understanding of the wisdom embedded in the premade Kundalini Yoga sequences.

> Once you begin to really truly understand all the elements [...] you know why those elements are in there.

Tanya's practice exists in sections of time sliced by the chimes of a meditation app. The pre-set building blocks of practice described above fit together according to the clearly arising intuition of the moment. Here the practice is a series of programmes with discrete functions to elevate lived experience and boost (inter)personal evolution. Each precisely timed block is bracketed by more mundane moments, spent checking notes and resetting the timer.

And yet within those pre-set blocks the emergent needs of the body make themselves known. In some long holds, a weakening body needs to be readjusted. Coughs disrupt the long periods of breath of fire. To pause, to weaken, or rearrange one's grip, as in Figures 5.24 and 5.25, is an accepted part of the lived reality of the practice. Tanya maintains her equanimity between external targets and the reality of constant compromise. To her,

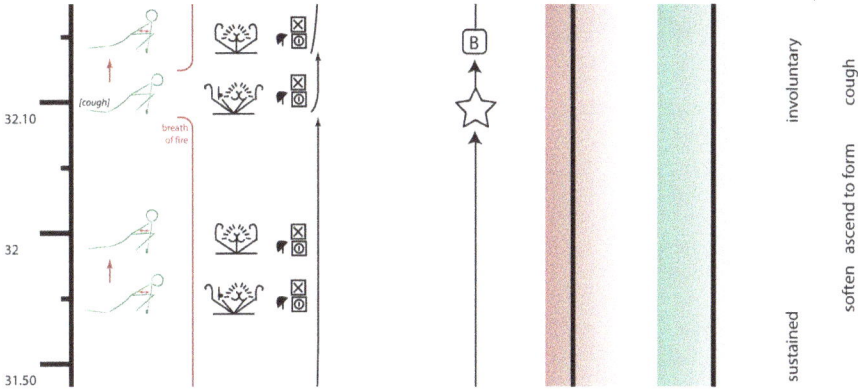

Figure 5.24
A moment to readjust

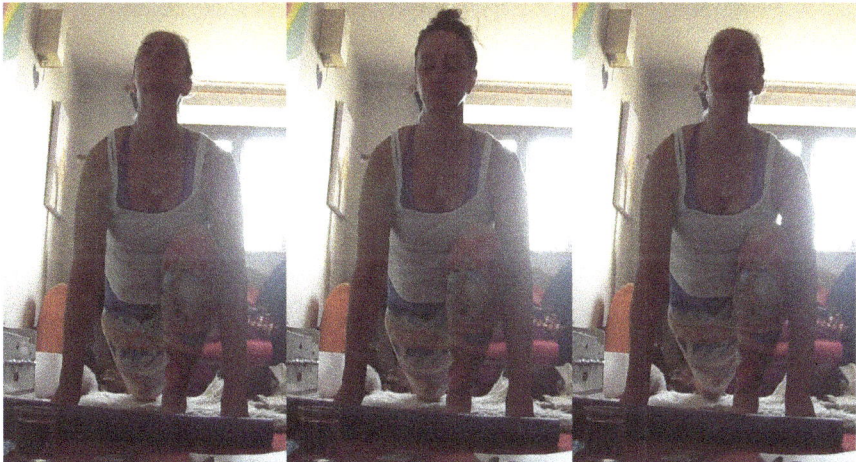

Figure 5.25
A moment to readjust

we are perfect souls imperfectly manifested, following each other on the slow path to greater realised perfection.

INTENTIONS AND OUTCOMES

Whether reducing addictive patterns of behaviour or increasing intuition, Tanya's practice intentions are concerned with changing the lived behaviour of the individual, framed within a humanist hermeneutic that focuses on our relationships with others. The relationship between researcher and researched is more evident here than in any other case study. Tanya explains her intent and clarifies points of internal processes to me between each block of practice:

> So just so that you know, because this is a really lovely practice. When you come up, the arms are spread like this, and then it's as if you're a flower reaching for the sun.

Despite many material additions to the practice space, for Tanya all space is equal. Field, canvas, brick and mortar are unified within a field of vibration, in which crystals and other objects are tools to a purpose, while the gods, spirits and humans, move with agency:

> You're invoking that energy [because] you've sat in there for years [...]. But energy is energy.

Tanya's yoga has always been shaped by the beings she has shared it with, since taking her mother to their first yoga class as a teenager. For her we learn through reflecting each other. Within that relational matrix, Tanya maintains a distinctly pre-modern epistemology. The Kundalini Yoga method works 'on the ten bodies, [...] the neutral, the positive, the negative mind, [...] the *cakra*s, [and] the *nāḍī*s' of the energetic self. The practice is a sequenced technology of energetic actions, accompanied by a consistently repeated internal *mantra*.

Rising on the endless breath of fire is *Kuṇḍalinī* (liberatory) energy in the service of spiritual evolution. The resulting trance state is not ecstatic, but clearing, erasing *saṃskāra*s (imperfections). The physical functionality of movement exists within the larger functionality of the whole self, evolving from moment to moment within an energetic, interpersonal matrix.

The raising of *Kuṇḍalinī* energy within an internal matrix, and the physiological stimulation of the nervous system are identical in expression. The body is held in a series of what could be considered stress positions, clenching *bandha*s (body locks) and squeezing the belly and jaw while repeating internal *mantra*s a set number of times, as seen in Figure 5.26, in what might be considered to be a compulsive manner. Reminiscent of the latest researches into early postural yoga by Mallinson and Singleton (2017), *mantra* and meaning are forcefully inscribed onto either the energetic body, or the psychosomaticised memory of lived experience, depending on one's epistemological understanding. The former serves the

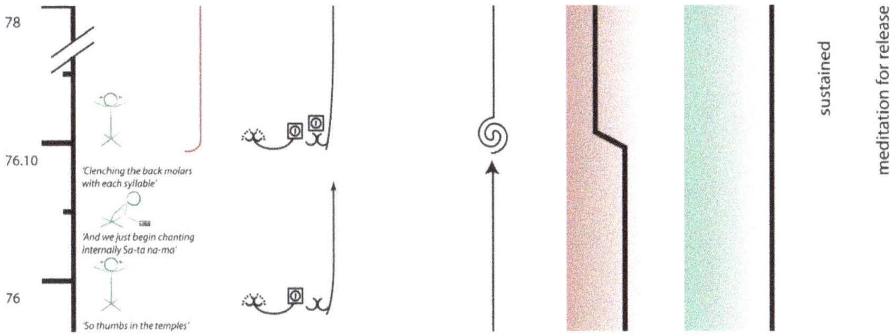

Figure 5.26
Clenching and pumping

evolution of the greater self, the latter could build either stress resilience or obsessive dependence on the method.

The clenching teeth, pumping breaths and held *bandha* (body locks) that are set components of the Kundalini Yoga practice, stand in opposition to the movement quality of soft bellies, eyes and tongues also common within post-lineage yoga. Yet any compulsive tension in Tanya's practice is released by moments of adjustment, rest and contemplation. The rising, drying fire of Kundalini Yoga meets the fluidity of post-lineage adaptation, and with the esoteric flow of fire and water, the nervous system may be tempered into steel. A sense of self-reliance is born of realising that every *kriyā* ends, every sensation passes. The raising, transforming and grounding of internal energies for the evolution of self-awareness is a common aim of these case studies. But this co-practice demonstrates how profoundly diverse the quality of that lived experience can be, even when exploring pre-set practice elements.

CASE STUDY 6

'One step in the world and one step in spirit'

NICOLE

When **Nicole** began her yoga journey, Iyengar Yoga was 'the only yoga in town', and for many years, that is what she studied, and taught. What she describes as the 'real rigour' of Iyengar, was supplemented by a later exploration of Ashtanga Yoga, again, as student and teacher. Both systems were important early steps on a long path that transcended both schools. Although she now develops beyond any lineage or school other than her own method, and states that the only authority over her practice is her 'internal awareness of energy', Nicole expresses modified respect for those who still defer to external authority.

Her own personal narrative describes a wild and possibly unsafe female body that encountered much-needed strict paternal alignment and discipline through Iyengar and Ashtanga Yoga. She then passed through multiple yoga schools, each of them conferring different physical or esoteric gifts, leading to growing intuition and self-reliance. It is, once again, a familiar story within the wider post-lineage subculture.

Nicole's most significant influence today is the founder of the more obscure school of **Shadow Yoga**, Shandor Ramete (see http://shadowyoga.com). Shadow Yoga is characterised by non-linearity and a fluidity of movement with strength more familiar from martial arts than yoga. Shadow Yoga practitioners are encouraged to individualise the system as it is taught to them, and eventually expected to develop their own personalised *āsana* sequences for their own practice and teaching. As I will show, Nicole's co-practice is an unusual one as a result.

Nicole's love of the more esoteric and internally transformative aspects of contemporary yoga also combines with a number of 'shamanic' trainings external to yoga culture. Her definition of this work hovers between the conception of emplaced negotiations with other than human beings common to the descriptions of many indigenous peoples, and the modern interpretation of core shamanism as internal healing through archetypes.

Nicole – Friday 27th May 2016, Bristol

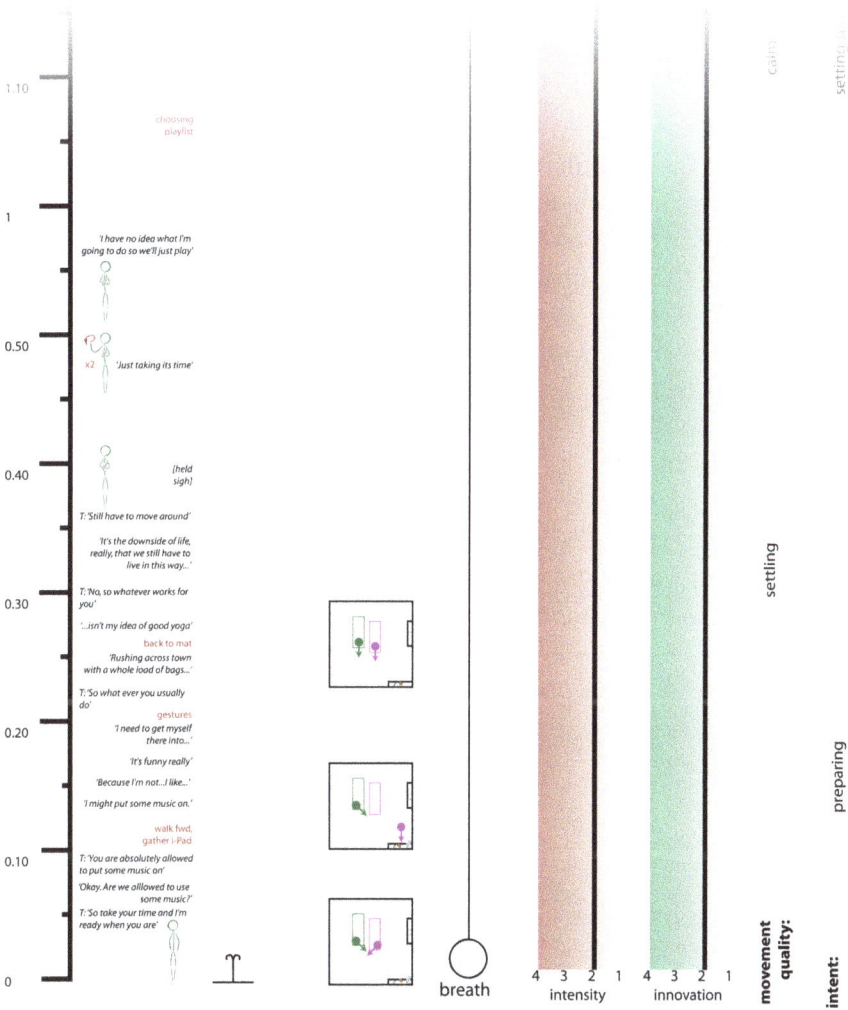

Figure 5.27
'One step in the world and one step in spirit'

Her eclectic practice sources culminate in her own style, which she calls Soma Yoga. It is the innovative nature of that style, as well as her long history and multiple connections within the subculture, which led me to approach her first at Santosa. Spiced with the hypnotic cadences and unusual paraphernalia of her shamanic practice, Nicole tailors esoteric and folkloric fragments from South Asian, Celtic and South American cultures to fit woven narratives of healing for self and a more than human world (Aarons 2017). Her radical syncretism resonates with her own multi-cultural heritage.

Over time, some teachers become so unique that they are largely inimitable, even as they, like Nicole, begin training other teachers in their methods. Taking trainings with them is not the initiation into an organisational hierarchy and affiliation to a set and systematised practice common to most modern yoga brands. It is more about learning *their* practice in order to see if there are elements one would wish to incorporate into one's own. As a result, forms proliferate, most teachers combine a small number of influences into their own blend, and practitioners attend post-lineage events to explore not just different ways of practising, but the different worldviews, and diverse personal histories inherent in each teacher's practice.

Despite decades of experience as both practitioner and teacher, Nicole claims enduring surprise when new students seek her out, and feels herself unsuited to commercial success. Like many of my respondents, Nicole is much more comfortable talking of specific, long-standing 'kinship' relationships than professional ones. She teaches at Colourfest, Santosa and Sundara, and speaks fondly of Christopher (Case study 2), Uma (Case study 3) and others who are key figures in local post-lineage yoga transmission.

Of all the case studies, she embodies one impossible ideal of post-lineage yoga: that of separating from the mundane and commercial world. Beyond her courses and sporadic Facebook updates, her media and social media presence is minimal, and includes such updates as:

> The winds of change are blowing us along new currents and we feel it in our sacred, secret beautiful heart. We need a maker of islands to hold us safe and offer us refuge.
>
> (Aarons 2017)

LINEAGE AND AUTHORITY

I meet Nicole at a yoga studio in Bristol, where she is later leading a workshop that includes *āsana*, meditation and *mantra*, but also a South American tobacco pipe ritual. For the co-practice we are alone in the quiet, empty studio. We aim for, and complete, a practice that is exactly 45-minutes long, despite not having a visible clock in the space. The session feels outside of mundane time, yet contained and held by it.

Nicole's practice that day is internally focused, yet without extended periods of seated contemplation. The metaphysical framework of the practice conforms to common subcultural associations of elemental symbolism familiar from Uma and other case studies, and with a complex, but long-established history in yoga thought (White 1984: 43). But the exact intent of each movement in this individual practice is so internal, and its expression so fluid, that it can be difficult to precisely confirm before the interview. Rarely does a single body part lead. Instead fingers curl into specific *mudrā*s to seal a particular effect. There are few repeated refrains in the *āsana*s, but the quality of movement is consistent and poised, particularly the early sections of the practice seen in Figure 5.28 which are generally symmetrical. Elegance is enhanced by Nicole's small but long limbed, extremely mobile frame.

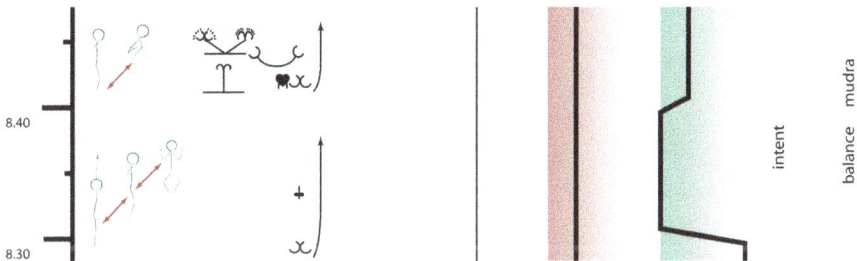

Figure 5.28
Symmetrical postures

This is a practice seeking balance in the energetic relationships of the esoteric self and surrounding space. Nicole moves fluidly through *āsana*s and Kundalini Yoga *kriyā*s, while using specific breath patterns to slide from one state of mild trance to another. The intensity of the practice rises and falls again in a series of steady waves.

Nicole includes a side lunging flow sequence similar to Christopher's (Case study 2), and a non-linear Shadow Yoga sequence (Figure 5.29).

Her Kundalini Yoga training is adapted to charge or release esoteric energies in specific ways. At various points, she employs the forced exhale of a *kapālabhātī* breathing practice, and a version of *ujjayi* breath with an open-mouthed exhale to release energy downwards, as well as the pumping breath of fire to lift or increase vitality. Each of these is adapted from the orthodox versions, lifted out of set sequences or performed in a non-standard *āsana*. Explaining the day's practice, Nicole says:

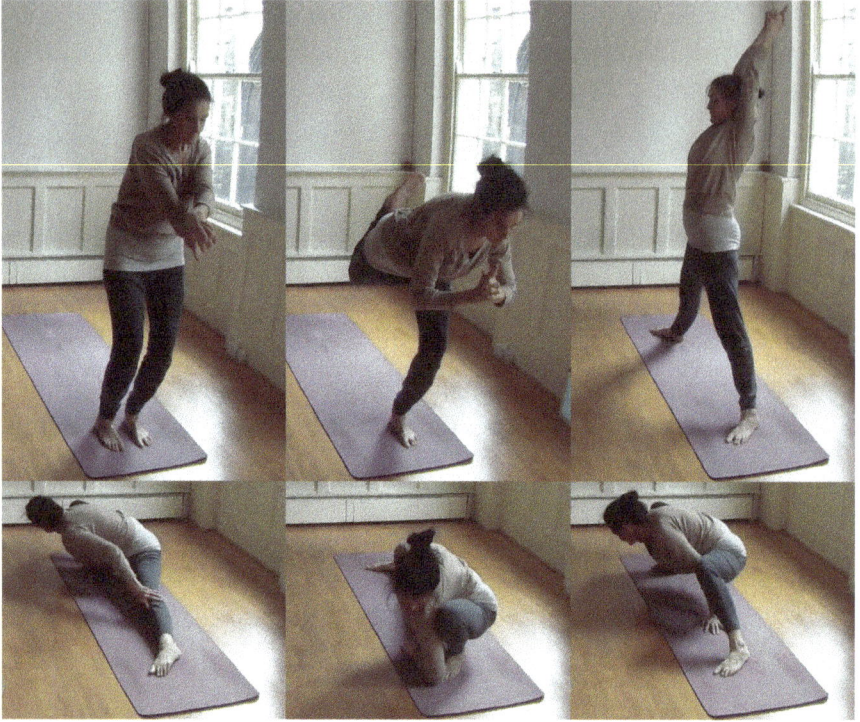

Figure 5.29
Non-linear elements

> Some of [the movement] needed to be slow, because I couldn't quite move the energy. And then [...] I sometimes did some more intense kind of *kriyā*-like movements to release it.

For Nicole her yoga is also consistent with her shamanic training and practice, because it brings in: 'a sense of sacred and ceremony.' She performs a lot of the practice with eyes closed, processing and transforming esoteric energies that she feels have accumulated either in dreams or the events of the day, and relying on her kinetic senses. Nicole also has an affinity with *yoganidrā* and lucid dreaming as described by LaBerge (1985), saying of her future practice: 'If there's anywhere I'm travelling, I'm going that way.'

She credits her shamanic practice with rendering fluid her personal history as well as personal geography, leaving her unsure of how long she's been teaching (over 25 years), or even her age: 'I've lost a sense of time in a linear way.'

Shamanic intuition renders visible patterns beneath the everyday that help Nicole to navigate this non-linearity. Nicole sees 'medicine wheels everywhere'. Just as Uma's practice visits each element in turn, and Sivani Mata's turns to ritually meet the points of the compass, her *āsana* practice moves to each of the four directions of a South American medicine wheel.

A number of the shapes described by Nicole's body in *āsana* are curved or spiralled, or trace one of her favourite symbols, the mathematical infinity sign. Symbolism is also bodily encoded through *mudrā*: hand gestures for different metaphysical elements, and the sub-culturally common '*yoni mudrā*', used to signify generative life force in nature. Just as her fingers hold to a shifting series of precise *mudrā* positions, so Nicole's tongue is placed or rolled across different parts of the upper palate, in an innovated echo of traditional *haṭhayoga* practices. The practice evolves through intuition rather than deliberation.

As an online article by Birney (2016) speculates, many yoga teachers in the wider transnational yoga culture are innately hypermobile, and so is Nicole, as we can see in Figure 5.30. She failed her Iyengar teaching exams twice for being 'too flexible', and she credits later practices of internal awareness for helping her learn to be strong enough to mitigate this tendency. As her physical rigour increased, so deepened her study of metaphysics. And that esoteric ecology provides a shorthand for describing somatic changes.

The Kundalini [Yoga] was good, I gained a lot of core fire [strength]. I never had a lot of fire. I had a lot of air. A lot of space. A lot of water. Not much earth and not much fire. So I've had to develop those things.

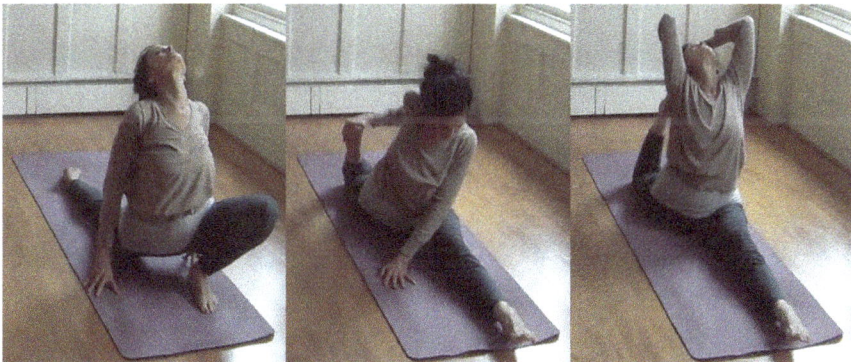

Figure 5.30
Working with hypermobility

Within the practice, *kriyās* and *āsana* sequences shift and transform esoteric energy, while *mudrās* and *prāṇāyāma* practices channel that energy.
Nicole begins each day and practice with raising her *agni*: her digestive
fire. Within our co-practice, that digesting fire is drawn through the body
sequentially:

> I'm creating fire in my belly, in my heart and in my third eye in order for me
> to digest things on those levels.

The practice ends at the point that Nicole feels entirely 'cooked', a state
which she describes as a 'constant balance of energies', free of any emotional or physical sensation that could be experienced as distorting the
flow between intent and action. This may be close to Veronika's equanimity in Case study 1, or Sivani Mata's place of balance in Case study 4,
although her framing points to a state different again from the former's
gentle frugality or the latter's abundant oasis. Like them, having checked
the inner landscape of the self for obstructions and distortions, Nicole
'can spend the day having one step in the world and one step in spirit
without feeling and being pulled in any one direction'.

For Nicole, inner landscapes reflect, affect, and are affected by external ones. While she has a dedicated space at home, with an altar that she
always returns to, she is at home wherever she teaches, and 'can practise
anywhere these days'. She contrasts this with her need to keep a 'consistent space' around her when she first began yoga. While her reactivity to
the immediate ecology of the practice may have diminished, her sensitivity to it has not. She describes arriving at the studio for our practice and
feeling 'the energies of a lot of other people'. She says later that the 'room
was not settled', blurring the boundary between herself and the space.

Nicole voices a statement I have heard from many practitioners: that
over time, less practice is needed to gain the same results. And as her practice has developed to be more achievable in energetically uncomfortable
spaces, so Nicole feels she has gained the power to change her immediate
energetic ecology through the practice. She is evidently much more settled by the end of the practice.

Nicole's disconnect from the mundane world and preference for intimate ecological negotiation are reflected in her ambivalence to wider
yoga culture. As a teacher who firmly positions herself on the edges of
even post-lineage yoga as a subculture, Nicole is yet clear that even personal evolution is delivered through a combination of 'years of practice'
and relationships with other people. Echoing Christopher, she says:

Guru is a process. Guru is a community. Guru is not an individual and it's not something that's ever fixed in time and space. How could it be?

INTENTIONS AND OUTCOMES

Nicole's practice, like others, is a search for balance in which the boundaries between the physical and the energetic, the internal and the external, become porous. The result, as seen above, is a unique iteration of post-lineage practice. Like others, her skillset has been gathered from a range of sources, in a long history of individual practice. She, like others, offers no shortcuts to this extensive, individualised learning process. There are occasional moments in our interview which are almost hagiographic, including her insistence never to have been injured, nor missed a single day of practice since she began.

This self-narrativisation is poetic rather than strictly logical, of a piece with the hypnotic way she leads students. But her desire for genuine, and generous relationship is clear. Nicole's identity is performed and reformed through her daily practice. In it can be traced the tension between her connection to post-lineage subculture, and her pervasive sense of difference from others. She dances gracefully through the quiet studio space with her own history, her unique morphology, but also with myself and the space as equally unique practice partners.

I am consistently aware of the different ways her body can move, as an invitation she is making back to my own uniqueness. Her favourite *āsana* is bound lotus (see Figure 5.31), which she can achieve without preparation, but which her students might never attempt. The practice she teaches is much more accessible, but there is a contained and charismatic ethereality to those sessions in which her unusual morphology combines with practised, graceful movement, hypnotic storytelling and esoteric knowledge to create a space that feels like a magical invitation.

Nicole's practice enacts her separation from the mundane world: from time, from geography, even at times from human biomechanics. Despite her modest awareness of her own popularity within the subculture, I found myself asking how much of Nicole's identity is cultivated, and how much a response to experiences, and how performative was the process of self-development? With all of my respondents, personal and professional identities meet, merge and are deliberately reformed in the process of practice. As we shall see in the following chapters, they are no less real as a result.

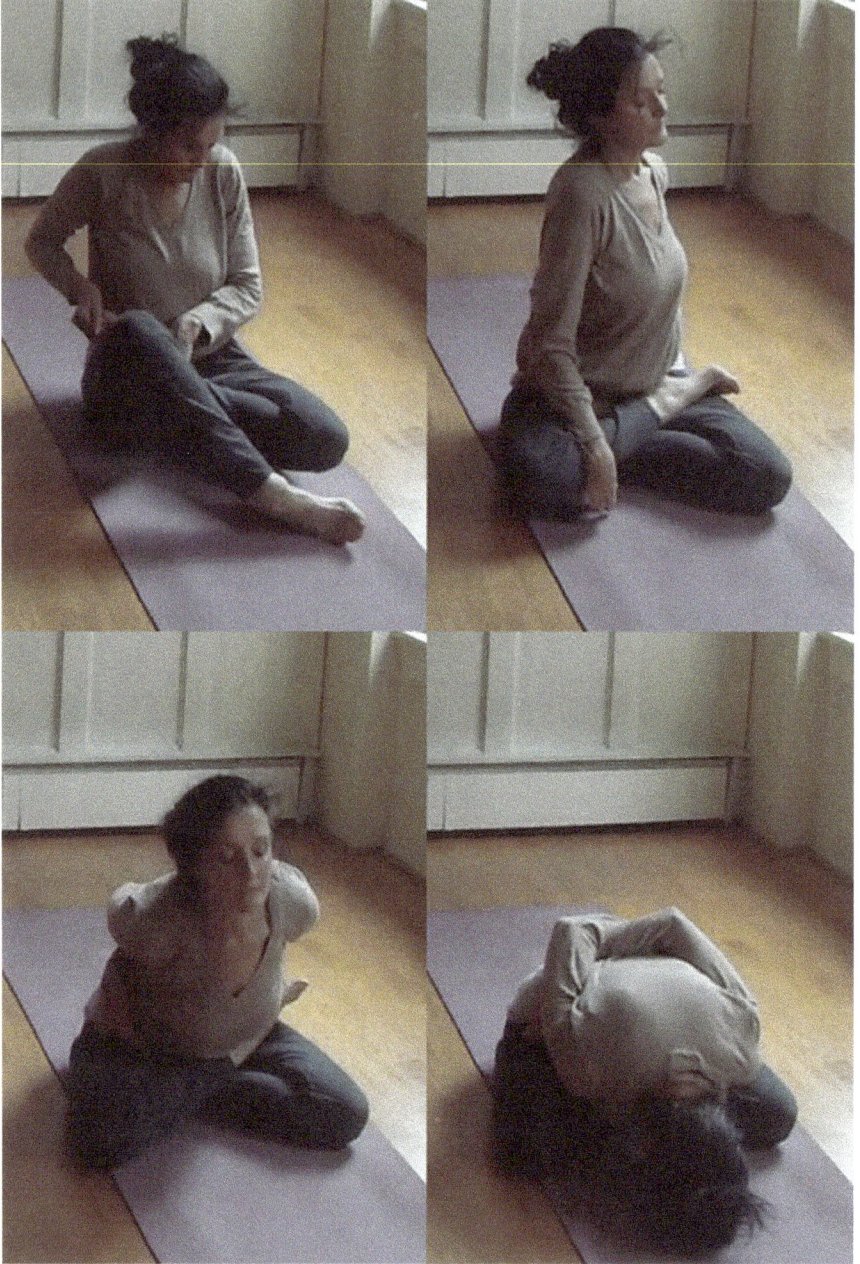

Figure 5.31
Bound lotus

CONCLUSION

Through the first case study, with Veronika, I have shown the common conception that practice is a balance between incremental self-transformation and equanimity. Hers is the first of multiple visions of a reclamation or evolution to a pristine state of being, somehow both somatically remembered and logically unimaginable. In this case study, I also showed her faith in both the gift of human self-awareness, and her love of all (animate) things.

Christopher's practice in Case study 2 is a process of self-maintenance, seeking the most appropriate response to a challenging world. His is a scientific animism of the body: what he refers to as a 'microbial inner temple'. In his case study I delineated two themes to question further: the implications of a disconnect between practice as it appears and as it is experienced for both research and teacher-student relations; and the marks of invisible authority left by a practice history, shown in the invisible yoga mat as a boundary for practice. Is truly spontaneous movement possible, given the ingrained habits of an individual?

The map for Uma's understanding of her abundant practice repertoire in Case study 3, is based in commonly understood elemental metaphysics, and her practice surroundings have agency as well as influence on the practice. Repeated practice with those metaphysical qualities, as a kind of experiential mnemonics, functions to re-pattern the somatic body. It renders into flesh subcultural metaphors such as waves of movement or lunar and menstrual metaphysics. The ability to call into being and embody such metaphors at will confers both personal empowerment and charisma in teaching situations.

Sivani Mata's practice in Case study 4 renders her own devotion to self and land more explicit still, through layered and repeated gestures of ritual that are both intuited and learnt. This case study outlined a number of productive tensions between purification and nourishment, inside and outside, lineage and inspiration. Here we also encounter the useful metaphor of practice as a healing oasis, in which arises a ritualised identification of self with other, world and deity.

Tanya in Case study 5 showed a very different practice. It combines Veronika's ontological humanism with the clearest influence of Kundalini Yoga and New Age esoteric understandings. This is a distinctly non-secular, yet supra-rational practice. Here, individual practice is a modular programme based on intuited choices from among the pre-existing wisdom of others.

Case study 6 with Nicole returned to many of these themes, from metaphysical energies, to the pristine self and the enduring balance between external authority and self-reliance. She stated most clearly the long-term benefits of individual practice and the lack of possible short-cuts. This case study further showed how otherworldly personal qualities can be managed and cultivated by practice, forming the conscious or unconscious basis for charismatic teaching.

The themes of intention and outcome drawn out of each individual case study are closely linked to themes already found in the communal practices shared at post-lineage events. In both settings, a series of productive tensions are emerging, across the borders between self and other, authority and intuition, and between enhanced awareness, increased equanimity, and effective change. To understand the purpose and processes of managing these tensions, it is necessary now to turn to the common framework underpinning such diverse individual practices.

PART III

POST-LINEAGE PRACTICE, CULTURE AND COMMUNITY

6

The construction
of practice

Despite numerous common inspirations for their practice, each of the case studies in this book is unique. Determining the commonalities and differences between any post-lineage practice and any other yoga practice is also complicated by the near absence of prior research into this, the (near) daily allegiance to a regular, ritualised practice of movement and stillness. Common connections can however be found between movement and intention. Just as in the group practices described earlier, in the case studies we also find effortful practices being seen as more 'masculine', and pumping breaths being linked with transformational aims. When this subculture talks about 'nourishing' practices, it is describing those that entail less effort and more rest. 'Devotion' is demonstrated through variations of physical prostration. 'Discipline' is practised through holds, repetitions and muscular engagement, as in Tanya's practice in Case study 5 (Figure 6.1).

'Freedom' and 'liberation' are experienced through mobility, as in Nicole's deepening backbend in Case study 6 (Figure 6.2). These broadly conform to the findings of Lakoff and Johnson, whose ground breaking research uncovered the physicality embedded in both everyday language and abstract thought (1999: 45–50).

The practitioner is able to create an individualised practice, which is expressed through a performance language created from shared practice elements with shared metaphysical reference points. Each practitioner constructs a personalised remedy for every condition, and a training protocol for every human quality. Sometimes practice reaches for an external ideal for the body or its behaviours to align with, and involves the

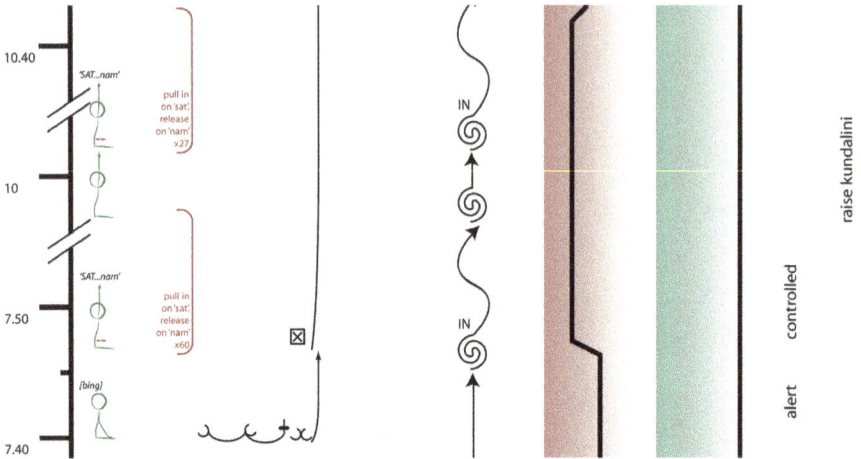

Figure 6.1
Case study 5: Practising discipline

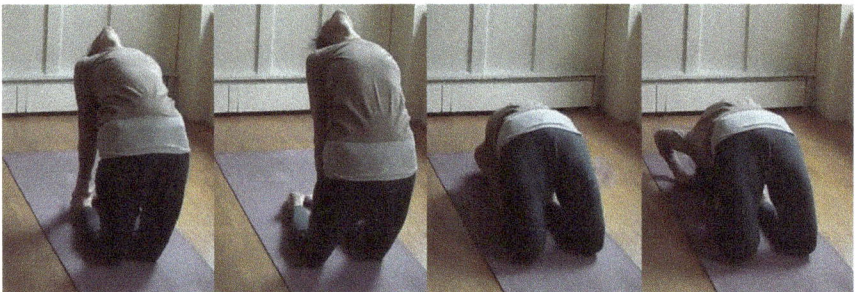

Figure 6.2
Case study 6: Exploring freedom

internalisation of ideal forms and movements. Individual practice that holds this intention to perfect is a process of self-correction, consistent with personal habitus, and the cultural distribution of biopower (Coleman and Grove 2009: 490; Lizardo 2004). Veronika's and Christopher's practices show this tendency most clearly in Case studies 1 and 2.

Sometimes practice appeals more to the somatic self, reaching for 'natural' or 'authentic' experiences. When this intention is invoked, self-practice develops proprioceptive and interoceptive sensitivity. The self-awareness that results is more phenomenological in nature. Meaning is found through the lived experience and intimacy of body and world. Those practising with this intention would agree with Bruno Latour that the body is a 'dynamic trajectory by which we learn to register and become sensitive to what the world is made of' (2004: 206). Uma's and Sivani Mata's practices show this tendency most clearly in Case studies 3 and 4.

For others, the practice has more esoteric aims. It involves the repetition of formulas of shape, sound and intention to pattern the physical self according to an ideal energetic body, or resonate in harmony with energies believed to be of divine origin. Post-lineage yoga breaks with those forms of early modern postural yoga which intended to create a Patanjalian body, impervious to the world (Burley 2014: 218). It is more strongly aligned with older yogic traditions in working with the idea of a bodily microcosm that is open and interactive to the macrocosmic universe (White 2006: 12). Tanya's and Nicole's practices show this tendency most clearly in Case studies 5 and 6. In reality, many post-lineage practices bring together self-corrective, self-sensitising, and supernatural elements, blending these three approaches. Each practitioner holds faith with the practice as a process of self-awareness and self-nurture, with one eye firmly fixed on some ideal of a perfected self as an eventual goal.

NEGOTIATING AUTHORITY BETWEEN GROUP AND INDIVIDUAL PRACTICE

Within the day-to-day, moment-to-moment lived endeavour of individual practice, identities are practised, performed, analysed and explored, but they are no less real as a result. What is becoming clear is how each practice aims to manage a disconnect between a wild or unique present self, a perfected or pristine self, and surroundings that can be mundane and depleting, or authentic and nourishing. Through these evolving relationships, post-lineage yoga practitioners produce resilience and self-nourishment, hagiography and charisma, and above all, newly authentic narratives of the self to be celebrated by the wider subculture.

Every *interpersonal* aspect of post-lineage yoga depends upon the generative power of regular *intrapersonal* practice. When teaching, it is possible for a single teacher to be responsible for choosing the intent and form of practice for a whole group of students. When those sequences of practice become formalised into prescribed routines for lone students to practise at home, each practitioner carries that deference to external authority into their regular individual practice, shadowing the movements and rhythms they have learned by rote. In theory, this is the method by which modern postural yoga lineages and brands reproduce themselves: increasing the number of practitioners while maintaining a centrally controlled uniformity for the intentions, outputs and form of practice.

But within post-lineage practice, that hierarchy of knowledge is largely disrupted. Thus, the *group* sessions of post-lineage events may be taught on a spectrum of more or less prescriptive instruction. But the *individual* practices of post-lineage yoga are without any single, external and above all stable authority determining the practice. In individual practice, the post-lineage practitioner may be repeating practice elements or sequences learnt from diverse, even contradictory teaching sources. They may be tailoring these elements for a better fit, creating hybrid forms, or innovating entirely new ones. All of these are subjected to verification with how the 'inner self' responds when practising alone, away from any group situation or teaching relationship.

The guiding authority during individual practice is not the guru or senior teacher, but a perfected avatar of the inner self of the practitioner. The goal of practice *is also* an incremental evolution towards that perfected or divine self. Such a perfected self is logically beyond the direct comprehension of the practitioner at the point of practice (Stirk 2015: 7). Yet the individual practitioner is able to partially imagine that perfected self into being, and cast herself forwards towards it, by asking her perfected self for guidance, experienced as feelings of ease or unease in the experiential moment of practice. Whether that final, perfected self can ever be realised is irrelevant. It is the use of the idea of the perfected self that enables the practitioner to explore and evolve within the instability of the self-at-present. That individual self is not only the final authority, but also the location, and the distant goal of practice, and freighted with the weight of personal history and expectation. In practice, this is as complicated as it sounds.

The many references to lineage, identity, intention and authority made in post-practice interviews demonstrate the centrality of this issue to developing and sustaining a post-lineage practice. Every moment as it is described is marked by both a deference to received wisdom, and intuited choices to be made by the individual in the absence of external authority. The ongoing evolution of individual practice is fuelled by such negotiations between the present self, the perfected self, and memories of diverse experiences as a student. Eventually, as I will show, the practice community will further ratify individually intuited practices, by adopting them into its shared repertoire.

Within the centralised knowledge hierarchies of brand and lineage, a practitioner might possibly innovate as part of their individual practice, but such innovations only translate into the shared repertoire of the practice community as a whole through narrow and officially sanctioned routes. In most cases, only the most senior teachers of modern postural yoga have the right to add to the shared repertoire of their school or lineage. In contrast, new forms of post-lineage practice are generated both in taught and individual practice, and above all in the relationship between them. Taught and individual practice are the two pillars of post-lineage yoga.

To the extent that each person, and each practice, diversifies authority beyond a single lineage or brand, one could expect very similar processes and themes to emerge in any post-lineage subculture. But there also exist other long and equally under-researched traditions of interoception and movement. Each of them depends on both group teaching and individual practice, each shares a similar urge towards introspective, holistic self-improvement, and each evolved with a diversity of more and less formal teaching hierarchies. From Dance Movement Psychotherapy to Body Mind Centring, it is possible that similar processes are applicable to many other such subcultures. As Kelly Mullan writes, for example:

> There are many gaps in the interrelated history of Western body–mind disciplines. It is only newly being recognised that there has been a growth of 200 years behind somatics, and 150 behind the growth of body psychotherapy. [...] While the approaches evolved and changed over time, the underlying philosophy has continually supported the 'whole person' as an integral being able to self-actualise.
>
> (Mullan 2014: 262–3)

In post-practice interviews all my case studies spent some time weaving coherent biographies for their practice, and linking themselves to well-known lineages such as Iyengar Yoga and Ashtanga Yoga, and less well-known, less hierarchical groups such as Shadow Yoga and Shakti Dance. Our discussions all centred around issues of authority, relationship, self-reliance, intention and practice. Questions immediately arose about the relationship of intention to lived experience. What is at stake, what is recovered, and what is elided by the emerging narrative of the performed, perfected self? In what ways is that self changed by the trace of other people on the learnt practice? What of the teacher is imprinted along with the practices taught?

All the case studies consider their practice to be devotional in some form, to the archetype of the guru and the gods, to life itself, to the spirits of the land, or to a potential perfected self, although none to a single, defined deity. The implications for each person's identity are profound. In individual practice identity is constantly re-forged through long-term, ritualised, visceral experiments in ontology. This movement eases one's breath, and thus one's connection to life. That bodily shape recalls another to the sensation of gravity in the body, and thus to the land beneath one's feet. This ritual washing recalls the profane and sacred nature of both self and teacher. All of these moments are in remembrance of, invocation to, and actualised steps towards a unique better self, and yet also resonant with a complex history of experience. The case studies show a deliberate porousness of the postural and metaphysical, the physical and esoteric, and of rational health to soteriological intentions.

AN INITIAL TYPOLOGY OF PRACTICE ELEMENTS

As I have stated, although there have been many attempts to categorise yoga practices, there exists no complete catalogue of yoga practice elements for either the pre-modern or modern period. Those schools that attempt this in the modern era, have done so most often according to the intention that the school has assigned to each practice element. Individual *āsanas* are grouped into categories such as 'hip openers' or 'backbends'. This is consistent with attempts to systemise *āsana* practice in particular into a therapeutic model, and is dependent on reducing each *āsana* to a single shape and primary intention.

My categorisation is based not on the diverse possible intentions or outcomes of each element, but on basic movement *qualities* that can be used to easily categorise *āsana*, and also the *kriyās*, *prāṇāyāma* and even *pūjās* common to post-lineage yoga in this particular subculture.

Each specific element from any part of the typology is chosen for practice, being emergent in the moment, intuited from prior practice, or the result of logical deduction. To become a regular part of a person's practice repertoire, elements pass through repetition into somatic memory, becoming implicit and primal. Such somatically embedded elements will re-emerge during later practices, as a response to associated stimuli.

Thus, a body scan will lead to particular results, that will be associated with particular choices about subsequent practice, and particular qualities of experience will provoke the body to habitual expressions of joy

Table 6.1 An initial typology of practice elements

Element type	Description	Breath	Variations (examples)
Pauses	Held shapes as a destination or series of stops within the flow of movement	Commonly held for multiple, sometimes counted numbers of breaths. Sometimes entered on a specific phase of the breath	Pauses held for a few breaths (*āsana*)
Pulsations	Rhythmic movements between two points.	Commonly in time with the breath	Metronomic movements to raise intensity (*kriyās*)
			Evolving movements to explore somatic responses (*pavanamuktāsana*)
Sequences	A series of emergent or pre-set movements that flow together	Conscious breathing, sometimes in time with movement	Recurring refrains of movement to warm, intensify intentions or allow for more automatic movement without the burden of choice (*vinyāsa*)
			Emergent or pre-set sequences with a single intent (hip opening)
Gestures	Movements of indication and invocation commonly made with the hands and/or head	Conscious breathing	Bowing and offering movements to externalised entities (*praṇam*)
			Gestures of the hand used to infuse and seal intent (*mudrās*)

Element type	Description	Breath	Variations (examples)
Adjustments	Movements external to deliberate practice	Conscious or mundane breathing, dependent on how external to the practice	Adjustments to clothing, props, or position in the room, eye contact
		Often expulsed exhalations	Releases of somatic tension (wriggling, shaking, sighing, joint adjustment)
Breath patterns	Specific breath patterns practised in any part of the practice	Specific breathing patterns	Rapid breath patterns that commonly enervate, sometimes practised in pulsations (breath of fire)
			Breath patterns that commonly calm, mostly practised in seated pauses (alternate nostril breathing)
Contemplations	Introspective practices almost always practised in seated or supine pauses	Slow, steady breathing	Seated contemplations (Vipassana meditation)
			Supine or prone practices of deep rest (*yoganidrā*)

or irritation. Finally, when a movement is fully embodied and embedded through practice, it can be re-embodied not only in response to certain conditions, but at will, with all its associations and experiential qualities, and taught to others. As I will show, when a teacher can model such a movement in that way, their teaching is more likely to be considered authentic by their contemporaries.

As an example, Veronika's body scan at the start of her practice in Case study 1, revealed a familiar tightness in her breath. In response, she chose practice elements that, for her, are logically and experientially associated with a sensation of release in that area of the body. Towards the end of the practice, having checked that her breath did indeed feel 'freer', she celebrated with movements that intensified the (now pleasant) sensations of the breath even further, and ended the practice savouring the somatic residue of those sensations, sitting in stillness. This specific connection of breath tightness to personalised remedy, is one that she can recall and model to others, allowing the subculture to determine the level to which it can be universally applied.

While this description may seem overly detailed, it is necessary to remember that practitioners themselves can struggle to articulate this largely intuitive process. It is also worth reflecting on the fact that this simple question: 'how do practitioners decide what to practise, and teachers know what to teach?' has not been the subject of serious study until now.

AUDIT, REMEDY, INNOVATE AND SAVOUR: A STRUCTURE FOR UNDERSTANDING PRACTICE CONSTRUCTION

All the case studies, and practices observed during fieldwork, contain most of the elements in the typology above. These are chosen as part of a four-part practice cycle: practices designed to audit the self; practices drawn from an existing repertoire; experimental forms, and finally practices of enjoyment (see Figure 6.3). Intuitively, all post-lineage practitioners learn to develop this spiralling technology of inquiry, contemplation, action and reflection in a cyclical process of unravelling and remaking of the self. The cycle is highly responsive, and for it to function well, practitioners must retain the authority to evolve and change elements, at least within their own repertoire for individual practice.

In this technology, consciously or not, they may have some commonalities with some pre-modern yogic practices (Mallinson and Singleton 2017: 7), but in their patterns of individualised authority they also closely echo other practices of self-reflection for self-improvement common to the European counterculture (Heelas 1993: 105), which overlap with bodily practices that exist in many cultures, but are exemplified most relevantly by a long history of European somatic practices, as mentioned above.

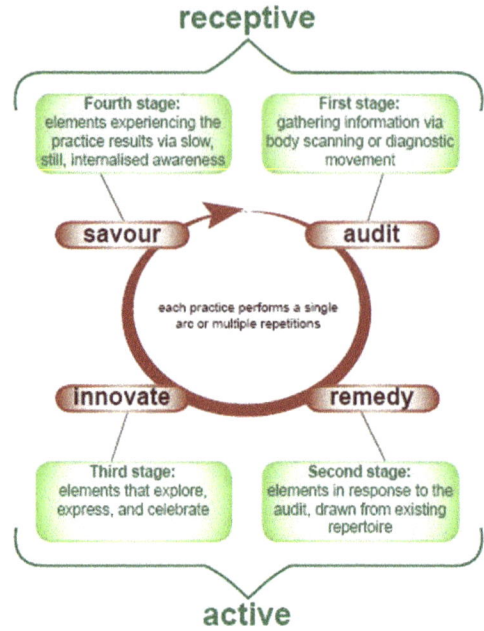

Figure 6.3
The practice cycle

Auditing the self

Above is a diagram of the practice cycle. In this model, the audit and remedy phases precede the more expressive and reflective stages of each practice. Both are dependent on pre-existing frameworks: the audit depends on pre-existing diagnostic tools and the remedy depends on a repertoire of practice. Almost universally, breath is considered to be the best adjunct tool for the auditing phase. As in most forms of contemporary yoga, breath is the interface here between body and mind. This may be reflective of known biology. There is an intimate connection between physiology, neurology and affect, governed and expressed by breath and heart-rate (Depraz 2008: 9). This connectivity was well understood within the pre-modern practice of yoga, as breath and life force are both included within the Sanskrit term *prāṇa* (Birch and Hargreaves 2015a). Thus, attention to the breath as a diagnostic tool enables investigation into all aspects of the body-mind and how they inter-relate.

Varying degrees of awareness or manipulation of the breath are associated with different neurological experiences. They are key to diverse practice aims. They are also reflective of often tacit understandings of what it is that a practitioner can feel moving with the breath, from the most physical to the most esoteric. In Case study 4, Sivani Mata talks about 'allowing the breath to move you'. Left unstated is a definition of the self that moves, or what can block its movement. A similar tacit understanding colours the following instruction from a Hatha Yoga session at Colourfest:

> Finding that nice balance in itself, so we can then meditate, breathe, without any tension or blockages.

In listening to practitioners talking about how the breath illuminates the body, revealing its potential for ease in stillness and movement, there is a sense of an inner landscape textured with somatic possibility and mobility that is remarkably reminiscent of Laban's descriptions of the kinesphere: the reach of possible movement that surrounds and interpenetrates the body of the dancer (Longstaff 1996: 21). For many of these practitioners, the kinesphere, the esoteric self and the porous body are all part of a continuum of experience. The physical self, the psychological self, and one's surroundings, all share such qualities as force and rigidity, softness and fluidity, heat, weight and dynamism. Exploring these mutual resonances, often in oppositions such as lightness and heaviness, empowers the practitioner to even greater depths of self-understanding and inter-penetration with the world (White 1984: 43). And yet bodily mapping is always more contingent, more conflicted, than this description suggests (Graziano 2016: 129). For practitioners, the unified self-world-experience is an enduring object of practice *precisely because* it is unstable and unverifiable.

Nonetheless, mind, body, world and spirit are connected 'metonymically rather than metaphorically.' (Alter 2006: 769). This means that they are porous categories of experience, in which practices for one, confer sympathetic magic to the rest. Thus, in one taught session alone, one *āsana* is named the 'cobra of wisdom', thought patterns 'dissolve with movement', and we stand on one leg in tree pose to mimic the 'tree of life'. In each case, the physical shape expressed by the body is more than evocative of its metaphysical associations. It instead expresses or calls such metaphysical elements into being. Each self-in-the-world is porous and evolving, yet coherent. It is helpful therefore to understand each practitioner, and each practice, as resonating with a particular configuration of self and world in a particular moment.

Accordingly, the right unifying narrative to frame one's experience is defined as the one that most resonates with as many aspects of the self and its world as possible. It can transform both the practice, and the self that practises (McHose and Frank 2006: 48). All of my case studies contain narratives in which the living self has an osmotic boundary drawn within a fluid world. Any edge drawn between self and divinity, self and surroundings, is a deliberate and temporary choice that allows for qualities to pass from one to another as a result of practice. Individual practice is a process that begins and ends with drawing a temporary, porous but coherent boundary to divide an outer from an inner ecology, and the true landscape of the self-world is a unified field of distributed qualities. Drawing a boundary around the inner ecology of the self, the heart of individual practice is an alchemical process that audits and then prescribes remedies to transmute heat into determination, fluidity into surrender, and so forth.

From yoga's inception, physical, psychological, spiritual and social benefits have been attributed interchangeably to practise elements (Mallinson and Singleton 2017). For this subculture, and in contemporary postural yoga more widely, intention aligns closely with epistemology, in that what can be reached for in practice is constrained by what can be known about the self through the body. Many of the conceptual maps of the self-world common to contemporary yoga come from disparate sources within South Asian traditions. These commonly include: Ayurvedic *doṣas* (Langford 2004: 4); Tantric *tattvas* (universal categories of energy and matter) (Mallinson and Singleton 2017: xix); Upanishadic *kośas* (layers of the self) (Mallinson and Singleton 2017: 184); and more modern, New Age interpretations of the *cakras* (energy nodes within the body) (Singleton 2010: 32). Detailing all the many ways that they have been adapted and transformed even within this subculture would be a worthwhile future research project in itself. But the use of multiple, even seemingly incompatible and unthinkingly overlaid maps of energetic and biomedical bodies onto individualised territories of lived experience serves a single function. When multiple maps from disparate sources can be made to interface with each other, they increase the possible field of 'routes' and 'destinations' within the self-world that post-lineage practice seeks to navigate.

This is clearest, again, in Veronika's practice, in which she uses the Anapana meditation from Vipassana, to decide the direction of travel of the subsequent physical *āsana*, the refrains for which are drawn from Ashtanga Yoga, but the detail of which is determined by Reflex Yoga. These practices originate from very different sources, and have probably been used together by no more than a handful of practitioners. But with them, Veronika is able to refine her practice until, over time:

Your observations go from being just what's on the surface or what's gross
or obviously sensation down to the much subtler things that are happening.
(Veronika, Case study 1)

This process of phenomenological inquiry provides knowledge of the
living self-world, the ideal self as it is filtered through current expectations, and the possible routes between them: the audit, and the remedy.
As a result, the long-term practitioner opens to what Veronika calls the
experiential 'universe inside you'. In passing, it is worth noting that the
use of infinity metaphors to describe the lived experience of the inner self
is widespread. It may reflect the ever-multiplying possible experiences of
the inner body. Or it may be that the indistinct nature of the interoceptive
sensory landscape compared with the more finite sensations of external
sensations on the skin, naturally recalls the numinous (Remski 2015b).

The most common long-term result of this kind of practice, as in
Veronika's case, is often described as increased equanimity. But each
practice, whether led or self-determined, is partly functional, partly diagnostic, partly expressive, and at least partly soteriological. And the multiple possible destinations of contemporary yoga, from healing trauma
to gaining material abundance and inching towards enlightenment, are
reached by multiple possible routes through the somatic inner landscape.
Any long-term post-lineage practitioner is expected to be adept at altering their route by adapting practice, and changing their destination, by
discovering new intentions.

To expand the field of possible destinations and routes, the practitioner's constant compass is the breath, and the *viveka* or inner discernment
that it enables. Intent and response are intimately connected during
practice. The maps of meaning that result are inspired by, and contribute
in turn to, the most common roadmaps of intent and action within the
wider subculture. Just as it is can be useful to think of religioning as a
process rather than religion as an entity (Nye 2000), so considering mapping as a contingent and dynamic process is more useful to understanding
post-lineage yoga than the multiple maps of its source material.

Practice repertoires as remedies

The second stage of the practice, the remedy, is dependent on an existing repertoire of shapes, textures and qualities that practitioners aim to
re-embody and individualise from shared subcultural practice elements.

As I have demonstrated, repeated practice with those elements creates experiential mnemonics to return to. Mapping practice and mapping the lived self includes both conforming to pre-existing norms and individualising innovation. The pre-existing repertoire and the process of self-auditing re-pattern each other in turn.

Intention, experience and expectation prime the body's somatic field and the resulting experience is coloured by pre-existing meanings. Even the possible intentions, experiences and expectations that frame practice are also formed from a lifetime of prior experience. Cultural narratives become solidified into the lived experience of the body in diverse ways (Bourdieu 1990: 68–69 in Lizardo 2004: 389). In mindful and self-empowered movement practices such as post-lineage yoga, those hidden processes of enculturation are made visible in a way that makes their disruption more possible.

How far the detailed correspondences of affect and gesture in practice are innate or learnt, tacit or revealed, is thus far impossible to say. Through incremental repetition, one person's gesture of communion can become another person's gesture of surrender. Through experiences of discomfort, one person's remedy for 'tight' hips can become another person's shape to avoid. Finding ways to map one's own sites of meaning and gestures of resistance within the individual body is in itself a lifelong goal of each practitioner.

The concept of repertoire I am using here implies a more self-conscious process than the predetermination of Bourdieu's habitus. It describes an evolving and self-empowered toolkit rather than a set of cultural givens. In many cases a resistance to habitus is a conscious intention of the post-lineage repertoire. This resistance may be effective to differing degrees. But among many others in the subculture, in Case study 2, Christopher practises at least with the overt *intention* to re-awaken the bodily universe in response to sensorimotor amnesia: the partial and uneven loss of bodily sensation and movement through trauma or disuse induced by contemporary living (Fraleigh 2000; Da'oud 1995: 349).

The intention of the early part of individual practice is to sensitise the lived body to both its habitus and the inner and outer ecology of practice, with an existing repertoire of tools. This is necessary before the practitioner can approach the spontaneity or communion hopefully discovered in the later moments of practice. In the long term, the nervous system is subject to increasing levels of refinement, and the motor capacities of the body are both differentiated and unified. In other words, the movement of the body becomes both more specific and thus precise, and also more coherent and thus graceful. Through the repertoire of remedy the practitioner seeks to return to a lived experience that is steady, enjoyable and graceful (Cole and Montero 2007: 303), and a body that is compliant to its own will yet also self-responsive to its needs. This awakened, actualising self can better discern the next step to the ideal self, can better surrender to the currents of experience, and can better navigate the sympathetic resonances in the fields of *prāṇa* and *kuṇḍalinī*.

Yet the very idea of repertoire and practitioner elides a further porosity of self to process. The lived self is not enacted *on* but *by* the practice. The experience of awakened, unified self-hood *is both the self and the practice*: a living sum of audit tools and repertoire, a landscape of somatic affect and gestures of expression that create the self that is expressed in the language of movement (Sheets-Johnstone 2010). As Stephen Cope describes it:

> In yoga it is understood that the experience of the abiding self is not so much discovered as it is created, moment to moment, in a field that is properly evocative, sustaining, and responsive.
>
> (Cope 1999: 137)

Thus each practitioner and practice balances achieving with experiencing (Haugen 2016: 79), giving weight to each dependent on their personal tendencies. Those seeking structural change strive for achievement. Those exploring phenomenological experience prize sensation. Aligned with that orientation is a correlating preference for either external action or internal homeostasis. Each action, however, increases homeostasis. And increased homeostasis makes action easier to perform. The resulting flow in each practice between action and homeostasis is visible in movement patterns.

In Figure 6.4, we can see the clear shapes of hand balances that Christopher uses to effect his intended action of strengthening the wrists. Between them are pauses to audit the results at 31.05, as well as shaking patterns at 31.15, which are commonly used in movement practices to reset the nervous system. Meanwhile Uma's practice throughout Case study 3, has a much stronger intention to experience homeostasis. It thus consists almost entirely of contemplative practices to audit and savour the self, together with emergent, wriggling and shaking movements that soothe the nervous system. Yet Uma's practice also involves minor intentions to address perceived imbalances in the body, and thus includes elbow-freeing pulsations and long-held stretches to 'open' the chest.

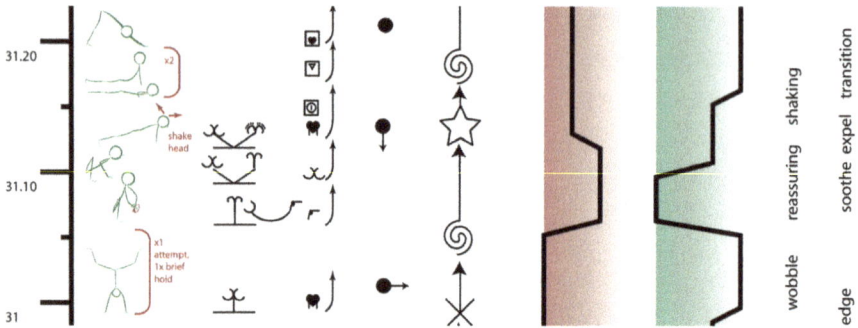

Figure 6.4
Case study 2: Pausing to audit and reset

It is instructive here to separate out choreographed action towards predetermined intent, from the emergent expression of bodily desires to shake and sigh. But in fact these are two poles of a continuum that echoes Uma's description of the necessary balance between *tapas* and *saṃtoṣa* as effort and ease. While a practitioner might tend to one pole or the other, each practice emerges in the dance between them. Practice changes the practitioner, and is productive of the meanings, as well as the selves it expresses. For example, esoteric *cakra*s are known to exist because they are a map of the body that correlates to the somatic experience of practice. Yet they are also installed through practice, called into being through repeated invocations of movement, sensation and meaning (Mallinson and Singleton 2017: 171). Post-lineage yoga is a highly **semiogenetic**, or meaning-making activity, in which many aspects of personhood are strongly implicated. It is a self-aware example of what LaMothe (2008: 583) calls 'a rhythm of bodily becoming'. Through this practice-as-repertoire, inside this fluid self-world, the self is a product and a process. The locus of intentionality, the self, is equally fluid.

In reality, there can be no self that pre-exists bodily experience. The proper term for the act and state of being-in-the-world, as Maxine Sheets-Johnstone reminds us (2009: 375), is not embodiment, but animation. Personhood is not installed in the body, but arises as a locus of concepts and actions, memories and processes (Ingold 2011: 11). Each of us arises from a field of sensation and movement that holds us enmeshed in our animate relations with the world that births us (Harvey 2006: 27; LaMothe 2015: 107). We are, indeed, inseparable from it, our porous borders continually reshaped by the relationships of consent, affect and action that connect us to others.

Savouring innovation and self-expression

For the practitioners in my case study, a lived experience of the emplaced, animate, evolving self as described above is a fundamental result of the practice. It commonly arrives in the savour portion of the practice, and it arrives wordlessly. It is not the fruit of the so-called primary senses of sight, sound, taste and smell, these discrete organs that seek to penetrate the world and return with impressions to be catalogued within the tidy corridors of the brain. Nor is it the result of reaching out to touch and change the world around them, or themselves to the world, ever-seeking Merleau-Ponty's 'maximal grip' on reality (Dreyfus 1996: 41). Instead, the implicit knowledge of one's place as an ever-arising, ever-connected, ever-ripening fruit of the world comes from those oft-forgotten processes at the heart of all experience: kinaesthesia and somaesthesia, in other words in the sensations of external and internal movement.

Regardless of the functional intentions to movement, post-lineage yoga overflows with an expressive surplus to functionality evident in both the innovate and savour parts of the practice cycle. This is maximal expression rather than maximal grip. Sivani Mata (Case study 4) and Nicole (Case study 6) in particular are adept at using the most internal of impulses to shape the most innovative and graceful flowing movements:

> then [I] feel into the fronts of the feet, I automatically feel the ripple and move from that ripple then I push through my hands and that ripples me the other way.

> (Sivani Mata)

If we consider the practice cycle on a qualitative rather than instrumental basis, every practice still builds from preparation to exploration, but often then moves to a number of peak, innovative moments that subsequent moments seek to savour. This echoes the arc of such ecstatic communions as the raves (Takahashi 2004: 155), dance and *bhakti* that are also strong influences within the post-lineage event environment. But the practice experience does not involve a simple rise to a peak followed by a single descent. It can be imagined as more of an octave of enchantment and intensity to be explored.

Trance experiences are not the sole reward for practice here. Long term practice can be as qualitatively mundane as it is ecstatic (Barsalou et al. 2005: 46). Most post-lineage practitioners in this subculture believe that reaching for peak experiences multiple times a week over many years is unsustainable. But each practice, and each interview, turned at some point to describe experiences of liminality and enchantment. The practice space is, in part, a re-enchantment of the sacred but mundane spaces of daily living (Holloway 2003: 1961), in which practitioners remember that 'we are at home and our relations are all around us' (Harvey 2006: 212). There is an experiential rightness to the practitioner during the savour stage of practice that reflects a resonant relationship with one's surroundings.

CONCLUSION

The distinction between sacred and mundane, though commonly made within the subculture, is both more complex and less dualist than it first appears. Among the many theological interpretations in this specific post-lineage subculture are diverse but common conceptions of remaking or recognising the bodily self as holy and invested with a spiritual, original self. This pristine self is sometimes described as separate from matter, but at other times, described as somatically silenced *within* matter. This deadening of the 'true' self is attributed to either the inevitable traumas of living or the dehumanising effect of contemporary culture. When, in Case study 6, Nicole describes living with 'one step in the world and one step in spirit', 'world' refers to a mundane experience of the everyday, and 'spirit' refers to an experience *of that same world* as enchanted and pristine. Thus, a practitioner who can walk in both is able to perform necessary everyday tasks *at the same time* as maintaining awareness of the miracle of existence: holistically united in experience.

In listening to practitioners talk, there is a strong sense of an intimate and sacred heart to identity. It arises in a process of self-divination within the oasis of practice just as, for some, the processes of cleansing and nourishment allow the *mūrti* to come into being during a *pūjā*. This self is named and called into being in a physical ritual of honouring, emplaced among an ecology filled with other *mūrti*s. Each *mūrti* is an incarnated, created version of something more universal, more abstract, more unified and perfected than the flawed incarnation that has survived to enter the practice. Within this enchanted space, the human practitioner is more than human. It embodies as many evolutionary and developmental forms as it can dream of, and every divine name it sings. It can be, depending on intent, both theomorphic and biomorphic (Da'oud 1997: 61).

The *siddhis* (supernatural rewards) of pre-modern yoga involved besting enemies and eliminating the restrictions of the mundane world (Mallinson and Singleton 2017: 361). When contemporary post-lineage yoga seeks the extraordinary, it dreams of creating a hyper-natural self that can maintain its awareness of both the mundane and the divine in all things, within a multiplicity of over-laid experiences. Thus individual practice is an 'intimate microcosmic self-sacrificial act' as Joseph Alter describes it, in which 'self, sacrifice, sacrificer, sacrifier and the ultimate object of the sacrifice all become the same thing' (2012: 426). The often-incommunicable state of enchantment that results is significant even and perhaps especially when it is not a prior intention, but an unexpected gift.

It becomes clear therefore that the 'inner self' that post-lineage practitioners refer to as the ultimate authority when choosing between the near-infinite options of possible practice elements, is in fact also the fuel, ground and eventual outcome of the practice. The relationship between the self that audits and the self that is audited, or the self that chooses and the self that is savoured, is an evolving mystery. The shift in authority that post-lineage yoga represents: from a single and clear hierarchy of knowledge to a fluid negotiation between the internal, external and relational, is further complicated by this practice cycle and its iterative evolution of the self-world as a landscape with porous boundaries. In the next chapter, I will outline the possible risks and rewards of such a complex, fluid practice, for a practice community that has differing levels of competence with the processes involved.

7
Teaching post-lineage yoga

Teaching the practice of yoga to others is at the heart of transmission within post-lineage, and indeed any modern incarnation of yoga. It is in the teaching of post-lineage yoga that this otherwise solitary practice gains its coherence and also its diversity, as it is unevenly translated from body to body, person to person. In pre-modern, modern postural, and post-lineage yoga, the authority to teach students also grants the authority to define the boundaries of what can be known, and what experiences can be held, within the practice of yoga. The impact of these changes in authority, and the importance of teaching methodologies in general, has often been underestimated. A brief history of what is known about the evolution of yoga teaching methods will allow the reader to understand at least some of the differences between pre-modern and modern yoga teaching, and thus better comprehend the development of post-lineage yoga. But this chapter should be read in light of the knowledge that, before now, the actual *teaching* of yoga has rarely been the subject of significant research.

RELATIONSHIPS OF AUTHORITY AND THE HISTORY OF YOGA TEACHING

In the pre-modern period, despite the existence of some manuscripts to support practice, most transmission of *haṭhayoga* was achieved directly between an individual student and teacher, known as *guru-śiṣya* teaching (Mallinson and Singleton 2017: 69). This is still held by traditionalists to be the gold standard for the authentic transmission of yoga. Practice was commonly transmitted via verbal instruction: the student is expected to do as the guru says, not mimic what the guru demonstrates. Furthermore, many pre-modern texts on yoga emphasise isolation as a condition of effective practice (Powell 2017). Therefore, despite the often intimate nature of the *guru-śiṣya* relationship, and in stark contrast to most contemporary practitioners, pre-modern students and disciples were largely expected to become competent through solitary experimentation, following personal guidance, but not under the eye of the guru in practice. In summary, then, the pre-modern era was characterised by one-to-one initiation and solitary experimentation, and depended on the spiritual authority of each guru over limited numbers of disciples.

As early modern teachers of yoga embraced group classes and an international sphere of influence, the exponential increase in numbers of devotees, and multiplying levels of teaching hierarchy, meant ever more power accrued to the guru at the head of most modern postural systems, while the common scepticism towards such 'god-men' largely failed to spread beyond India (Newcombe 2017: 19). The common Hindu idea that a person can gain spiritual benefit through direct presence with a more enlightened being, has continued to cast a shadow over the resulting interpersonal power dynamics whenever yoga practice is shared in group instruction.

In formulating new methods of teaching suitable for group classes, the modern renaissance of yoga also imported colonial pedagogies that included group instruction by rote, and corporal discipline. Most modern postural yoga teachers continue to use physical adjustment to enforce standardisation in anatomical alignment among students (Sarbacker 2014: 106). In contrast, post-lineage yoga teaching begins to question not just the hierarchy of knowledge among yoga teachers, but the authority of the teacher to decide the needs of the student. They are significantly less likely to correct or physically adjust students.

Of course, this description is a generalisation that highlights the differences rather than consistencies between pre-modern, modern postural and post-lineage teaching styles. It also does not tell us how effective each approach might be in achieving its aims. And rare forms of *haṭhayoga* persist that are taught in the traditional fashion (Smith 2008: 140). But in contrast to the advice of most pre-modern guides to practice, the teaching of modern postural yoga has been largely achieved via in-person group classes. This fundamental difference explains the lack of postural detail in pre-modern teaching compared to the extensive verbal instruction and physical adjustments included in most of modern postural yoga, which are often delivered as the student practises (Moore 2013; Hauser 2013b: 114–15).

The modern postural yoga teacher is an expert instructor, who issues detailed commands to groups of students according to universalised standards of correct posture and movement. Modern postural yoga teachers encourage students to develop a regular individual practice that reproduces the system as it is being taught to them, and, just as in individual practice, the teaching repertoire of modern postural yoga mostly consists of pre-set techniques drawn from only one named lineage or brand. Each school's teaching content is, therefore, a complete and discrete pedagogical system that determines both shared and individual practice in some detail. The authority of each practice lineage is transmitted over time in a hierarchy of knowledge: from recognised teachers, to a minority of students who are already regular practitioners and thus living libraries of practice, as they become teachers in turn. Where innovation in teaching *does* occur, it must be consistent with existing content, and ratified by the teaching hierarchy. And when new practice elements are added to the common repertoire, references to external sources are often obscured in preference for emphasising any coherence with existing practices.

In contrast, each post-lineage teacher's practice repertoire includes elements from a range of lineages, and even non-yoga practices. Post-lineage teachers are more often guides than they are instructors, facilitating a range of options for students to choose between. They are more likely to openly acknowledge diverse sources for their knowledge, mentioning articles they have read or workshops they have taken. They are also more likely to emphasise the newness or innovation of recent additions to their repertoires than any consistency with existing practice. And when encouraging students into a regular individual practice, post-lineage teachers are likely to stress the importance of developing *intuition* as well as of developing *discipline*.

This difference can be further illustrated by expanding a poetic metaphor used by Matthew Remski: that of the 'stonecutter and the baby whisperer' (2014b). Modern postural yoga teachers function like junior sculptors within a large studio, exposing the ideal form within each student body according to the instructions of an (absent) master craftsman. Post-lineage teachers are more like independent therapists, using a peer-agreed toolkit of techniques to coax the student body back to its own, innate wisdom.

The authority to determine practice has often rested with each teacher or guru, within fixed systems of knowledge, surveillance and authority. Post-lineage yoga does question many of the assumptions governing authority in modern postural yoga. But in many ways, the aura of authenticity that pervades the *guru-śiṣya* relationship continues to confer an invisible aura of mysticism and charismatic power onto all teacher-student relationships.

Many of the historical and ongoing changes in teaching practices are intimately connected to the rising ratio or at least visibility of female practitioners compared to male ones (Mallinson and Singleton 2017: 52; Singleton 2013: 51). Historical teachers from Indra Devi (Goldberg 2016b) to Vanda Scaravelli (1991) and contemporary teachers such as Angela Farmer (van Kooten 1997) and Uma Dinsmore-Tuli (2013b) have been at the forefront of many radical departures in yoga teaching methods. Many of them have attempted to shift authority from lineage to community, and from pedagogical control to inspiration and encouragement (Davies 2013: 42). More recent investigations into the biographies of such teachers reveals a common drive for that shift: their experiences of injury or ethical failings in lineage environments (Remski 2017). As Scaravelli wrote, rather optimistically:

> The worship of authority, of gurus, priests, teachers, is over. To question authority is the mark of a good mind, unafraid to explore.
> (Scaravelli 1991: 48)

Yet many of these prominent female teachers were also charismatic figures who inspired reverence if not deference in their students. Some women, including those featured in this book, have found in yoga a rare space to lead powerful rituals, and shepherd congregations of students. For some, contemporary yoga offers the opportunity to reclaim agency over their religious life as much as over their health (Aune 2011: 97; Westoby 2018). The role of both modern postural and post-lineage yoga teacher is therefore also a pastoral one. Not all abusive or injurious behaviour is carried out by charismatic male gurus within patriarchal lineage structures, however. Any injury received in the context of yoga practice can be attributed to any number of causes: a pre-existing weakness, a student not following instruction correctly, or a badly trained or over-confident teacher. Any emotional breakdown in the context of yoga practice can be explained as an ecstatic liberation, a necessary catharsis, or a pathological response to cultic manipulation. This can occur no matter who leads the process, or the size of the group, or the authority structure which legitimates it. Some criminal actions are the product of groups rather than leaders (Falk 2009: 137) and some abusive experiences are led by young, female teachers (Scofield 2018). Although less often than men, female yoga teachers have also been accused of financial, emotional and sexual abuse by their students and devotees (Tredwell 2013; Remski 2016b).

Modern postural yoga, in particular, is popular precisely because the promise of a series of set *āsanas* with confidently expressed universal benefits, which are selected in line with teacher-diagnosed needs, is attractive to a student body of casual practitioners, who are often both extremely anxious and somatically dissociative (Apperley, Jacobs and Jones 2014: 726; Lavrence and Lozanski 2014: 80). Modern postural yoga teaching techniques therefore most often aim to reassure students, to keep them feeling safe, to entice them from more popular to less accessible offerings, and above all to improve their wellbeing, often through the performance of universalised ideals of health, and standardised methods of instruction (Jain 2014a: 112).

Yet recent research suggests such biomechanical universality may be largely illusory (Gilman 2014: 63). Subjective experiences such as 'good' health, wellbeing and confident, self-aware movement are complex, socio-politically influenced phenomena (Lederman 2010: 10; Geeves et al. 2014: 682). Besides this, corrective instruction risks inducing adverse responses in which healthy ranges of movement actually become more restricted than before (Behnke 1997: 189; Tumminello and Silvernail 2017). And the large amount of detailed instructional stimuli delivered by many yoga teachers can itself enhance the possibility of reducing agency (Stirk 2015: xii), learning capacity (Junker 2013: 167; Goldberg 2016a: 402) and even a student's ability to perform as instructed (Kane 2018; Wulf 2013: 90).

Furthermore, despite the many changes in the teaching of yoga, few if any modern postural, or indeed post-lineage, yoga subcultures have developed a coherent teaching philosophy to underpin the mechanics of instructional techniques. Although there has been a rapid increase in all forms of yoga teacher training from the late twentieth century onwards, the emphasis in the majority of courses is on the *content* rather than the *reasons* for teaching protocols. This is often framed by the briefest of discussions of Patañjali's *yamas* and *niyamas*, pre-modern rules for right livelihood, which are a mandatory inclusion in teacher training curricula for most accreditation bodies (IYN 2018).

Examples of more robust and detailed ethical codes do exist, but as the explanation for one draft explains: 'the prevailing argument is that Patanjali's Yamas and Niyamas should be enough' (O'Sullivan 2017). Besides these, many yoga teaching bureaucracies struggle to agree on a scope of practice, code of ethics, or even agreement on which organisations or individuals would be consulted in creating them (Jain 2014a: 97). The kind of peer and mentor support structures so vital to many therapeutic professions are informal, and rare.

This situation is starting to change, but the changes implemented in the process are frequently controversial, as demonstrated by the often outraged responses to proposed National Occupational Standards for yoga in the UK (SkillsActive 2017; Remski 2016a). Within post-lineage yoga, as with every other aspect of the subculture, responses to the issue of standardisation are diverse, often innovative, and frequently individualised, but non-institutional solutions are always preferred. Many would agree with Vanda Scaravelli that 'yoga cannot be organized, must not be organized. Organisations kill work' (Scaravelli 1991: 68).

POST-LINEAGE INNOVATIONS IN TEACHING

Post-lineage yoga encompasses more diverse forms of instruction, just as it encourages a more diverse practice repertoire. But as shown earlier in this book, post-lineage individual practice is also an expression of each person's unique inner history. This increases a post-lineage yoga teacher's reluctance to universalise the practice when teaching others. Post-lineage yoga teachers are more likely to refrain from prescribing details of practice for students, and more likely to develop teaching methodologies that aim to incrementally improve each student's *own* ability to confidently navigate a wide practice repertoire, and encourage them to make choices in class and individual practice.

Many innovations in post-lineage instruction are therefore consistent with the principles of participatory education. These include four common changes from the modern postural teaching methods they were probably first trained in. Verbal instruction is more likely to be *invitational*, rather than imperative. *Choices* are given, with information to help students in choosing the right option for them. Teachers are less likely to say 'now do this', and more likely to say 'if you're feeling this way, you might want to choose this option'. Many of the options available are modifications that enhance the *accessibility* of a practice, for those with smaller ranges of motion, or whose body types struggle with *āsanas* that favour leaner, longer limbs. Finally, increasing numbers of teachers are also reconsidering their assumed right to adjust students, and experimenting with protocols of *consent* governing physical touch.

At the events featured in this book, it is assumed that all practices are accessible to all unless otherwise stated. The right to enter and leave a session at any time is universal. And many teachers are adopting the language and consent-to-touch protocols developed by Emerson and Hopper (2012), and Hala Khouri (2016), among numerous others (Jones 2017) within a loose collection of yoga forms that were first developed for those living with PTSD and still described as 'trauma-informed'. One session at Sundara is typical of 'trauma-informed' instruction:

> Perhaps keeping the hips lifted and then taking the arms by the side of the body. You can even, if you want to, walk the heels in a little more so you can feel that sense of lift. [...] Not pushing in an unkind way or uncomfortable way. Easing and listening. [...] Taking your time and noticing the sensations of the body.
>
> (Calma yoga session)

Trauma-informed yoga is of rising relevance, because of the growing use of yoga among other movement practices, for the management of PTSD and similar chronic conditions (Brom et al. 2017: 1; Compson 2014: 276). A number of post-lineage yoga teachers are involved in developing this therapeutic work, including the teacher quoted above. They aim to teach such students useful skills for neural self-regulation, and to improve intuitive decision-making in a population whose most significant common experience is a loss of control over life events (Van der Kolk 2014: 27). Such techniques are by no means exclusive to post-lineage yoga, but they are encouraged by a willingness to question prevailing orthopraxy, and an enthusiasm to develop significant internal authority over practice. Post-lineage teachers are thus more likely to be early adopters of both trauma-informed and accessible yoga techniques, in many cases putting them ahead of the curve of transnational yoga teaching norms.

Post-lineage teaching techniques include a number of other methods for devolving authority in group classes. Among the simplest, and most common, is the practice of teaching in a circle, where every student's visual attention is on the group, rather than in lines, where each student faces only the teacher (Sheets-Johnstone 2017: 16). These circles are echoed by a practice repertoire that more commonly includes circular and spiral movements. In group classes these pulsating or circular movements allow each student to repeat, innovate, and work at their own pace within the timing of the session. In the Chi Yoga session at Santosa that was discussed in Chapter 4 (Figure 7.1), circular movements of the ankles followed by rising and falling motions of the knees were instructed in time with the student's breath rhythm, but with little anatomical detail, leaving students to explore their own version of the movement.

"Chi Yoga" with Barry Elms - Shakti Ma dome, Santosa 7.30 - 9.30 pm Friday 26th Aug 16

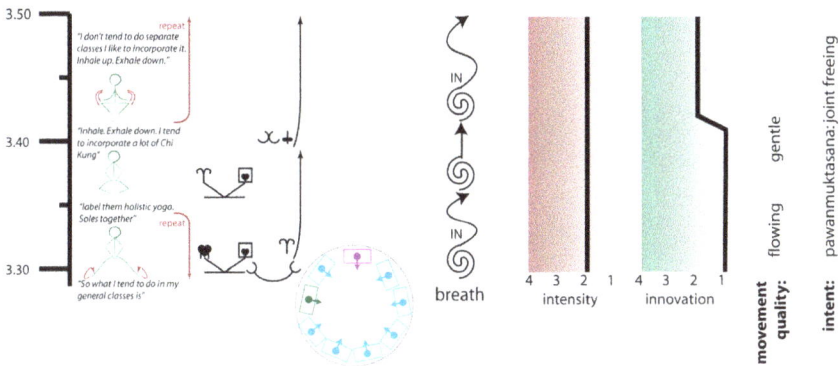

Figure 7.1
Santosa: Finding your own rhythm

In another Shakti Dance session at Colourfest, students moved to the unifying rhythm of pre-recorded music, but were asked to explore shapes in that movement as variations on a theme:

> They can go in spirals, they can go in open curtains ... Then going slowly. Lower. Around the solar plexus ... Imagine that there is a vortex, pulling out like a fan.

The emphasis in instructions thus moves away from achieving a set shape and then moving on at the teacher's next command. It becomes an internalised process of witnessing and experimenting consistent with the practice cycle set out in the previous chapter. If participants are arranged in a circle, that process of witnessing can be externalised to the group, as in this Authentic Movement session from Colourfest:

> We're going to invite any one of us, or two of us, to step into the middle and explore their dance while being witnessed. So, taking what you've

discovered already and allowing yourself to be seen and to be heard and to be met by the group.

More recently, collaborations between teachers are becoming increasingly popular at many of the events I have attended. These are not pre-planned in great detail, and are often experimental. Nevertheless, they also model the distribution of authority over practice to multiple people in the session, and students are able to appreciate the ways in which teaching is emergent and contingent on both place and participants.

The uneven translation of the practice cycle to group instruction

Like most contemporary yoga teachers, post-lineage teachers are life-long learners (Van der Zee 1996: 165). As such, they tend to continual self-development, embracing educational opportunities in an individualised and pragmatic manner. New teaching techniques are acquired in a piecemeal rather than systematic approach. Accordingly, translating the individual practice cycle described in the previous chapter into group teaching is unevenly achieved, in variable versions of the processes of *audit, remedy, innovate* and *savour*. Opportunities to *savour* the rewards of practice are included in the intentional and energetic arc of almost all sessions, in moments of silence and practices of more self-contained stillness, from meditations to relaxations to momentary pauses in restful poses. In contrast, the balance between the *audit* and *remedy* parts of the cycle varies significantly within each taught session.

As is widespread in modern postural yoga, some post-lineage teachers will still *audit* student needs on behalf of the group as a whole. Their instructions to students will focus therefore on prescribing *remedies* for those teacher-audited needs, and consist of three main types. Most common are anatomical cues that impose postural alignment, such as: 'place your hands on the mat, shoulder width apart'. These have their roots in group exercise, corrective therapy and military drills (Armstrong 1953: 236). These are sometimes accompanied by descriptions that assume all students will have the same result to practise, such as: 'lift your head and feel your heart expand with your breath'. Timing cues are also used to coordinate the students' breath and entrain the group to a common rhythm, such as: 'inhale and step backward, exhale and lower to the ground'. The challenge of all these instruction types is to map every

student's need effectively, and communicate any corrections or adjustments that can enhance the student's experience in a way that improves
both their practice, and their understanding of it (McIlwain and Sutton
2014: 657).

Figure 7.2 shows an example from a session at Sundara that retains a
number of the above elements, but also signs of more individualisation
and encouragement to student agency. To begin with, the teacher is
instructing the group as a whole in a held *āsana*. At the same time, she is
using her hands to guide a student's hip into what she considers to be a
more appropriate alignment. The teacher proceeds to instruct the class in
some detail in what she understands to be a universally safe process for
transition to the next pose, but invites them to move in time with their
own personal breath rate rather than a common rhythm. In the process,
two options are given for knee position to accommodate different levels of
flexibility. Here the extensive instruction is given so that the students can
be confident that they are moving as expected, and the teacher's narrative
style is more helpful than corrective, but an external and universal ideal

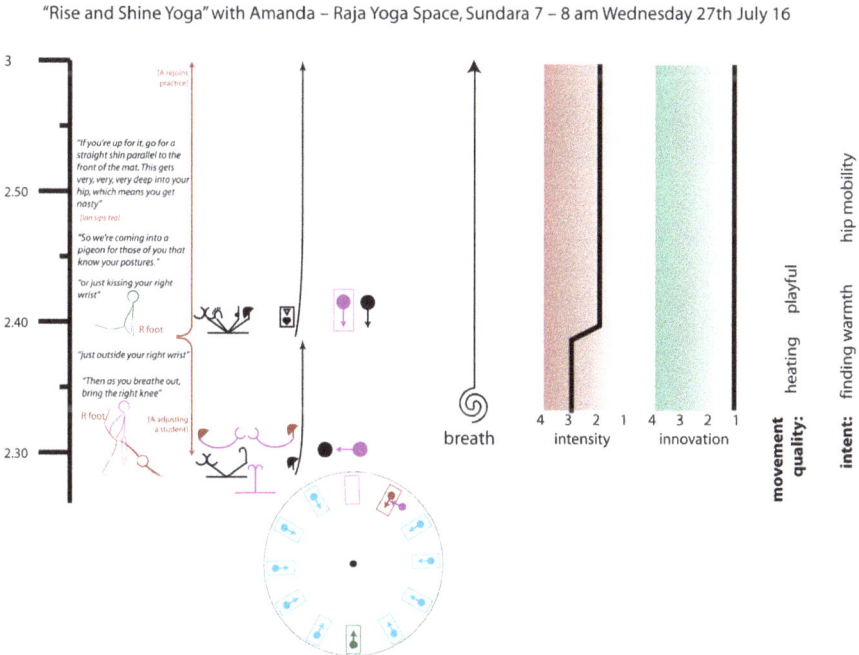

"Rise and Shine Yoga" with Amanda – Raja Yoga Space, Sundara 7 – 8 am Wednesday 27th July 16

Figure 7.2
Sundara: Combining correction and accessibility

is still in evidence. Finally, a universalised idea of what the new *āsana* will feel like to all is narrated by the teacher (in this case, irritable).

> Then as you breathe out, bring the right knee just outside your right wrist, or just kissing your right wrist. [...] If you're up for it, go for a straight shin parallel to the front of the mat. This gets very, very, very deep into your hip, which means you get nasty.
>
> (Rise and Shine Yoga session, Sundara)

Post-lineage teachers who are more influenced by hybrid and alternative knowledge bases, such as dance, Scaravelli Inspired Yoga, and the many divine feminine yoga schools, are more likely to concentrate their instruction on the *audit* phase of the cycle, and leave the choice of *remedy* more to the individual student. This type of teaching will consist mostly of cues and practices to improve awareness. Instructions are of three main types. There are cues to direct attention to specific parts or aspects of bodily experience, such as: 'bring your attention to the contact between your hands and the mat'. There are movement cues that will provide sensory input to enhance awareness, such as: 'as you lift your arms, notice if that changes your breath'. And there are multiple suggestions for various movements that might change the student's experience of the practice: 'you might like to come to the ground now, or stay here exploring your balance a while'.

Below is an example of instruction from a Scaravelli Inspired teacher at Colourfest. This extract is taken near the start of the session. The teacher's intention is to awaken the students' awareness and mobility of the feet. She directs their attention to their toes, and suggests that they 'might' want to lift them as a response to what they experience. Her instructions are highly invitational, with various options offered. Finally, she asks the group to follow the inner guidance of their imaginations for the session as a whole. The challenge for this kind of instruction is to develop student awareness in an environment of high entrainment and suggestibility:

> I'd like you to feel your toes in particular. So, the big toe, and then going across all the toes. You might feel you even want to pick them up and play with them a little bit. Give them a wiggle, a stretch. So, let your imagination guide your practice today.

While post-lineage yoga teachers will tend to the invitational or, more rarely, the prescriptive end of a spectrum, most will combine instruction styles. The least common part of the practice cycle to translate to a group environment is the *innovate* aspect, as it is much harder to set boundaries or create a unified experience when each student is following their own intuition. Those teachers with invitational instruction styles are the most comfortable holding a pedagogical space for the spontaneous movement involved in encouraging student experimentation.

However the cycle is translated from individual to group practice, it is the gaps in perfect transmission between each teacher and each student in terms of diverse biomechanics, exact movement, somatic experience, and frameworks of meaning applied to the experience of post-lineage practice that most enable innovation (Sutton 2011: 356). Indeed, similar slippages in understanding contribute to the evolution of shared repertoires of all kinds (Cuffari, Paolo and Jaegher 2015: 1121). In every session can be found multiple examples of how such gaps in transmission promote diversity in practice.

In Figure 7.3, we return to the 'Rise and Shine Yoga' notated in Figure 7.2. The photographic evidence shows that even when instructions are given to the whole group, the actions of each student can vary considerably. Here, some students are taking the various options given, but in the third image, the student who was adjusted takes a moment on hands and knees instead of coming to the next *āsana* directly, and one pauses while in the *āsana* to take a drink.

In another session at Colourfest, the teacher gave a series of simple instructions. Students were invited to take their prefered variation of headstand, to exit in their own time, and then to take up some version of the commonly practised 'child's pose'. Again, some took diverse variations of headstand and child's pose, transitioning from one *āsana* to another in various ways, and one being specifically assisted by the teacher. But others sat and watched or otherwise chose not to follow the instructions at that point. Even when movement is closely prescribed, there is a clear distinction between the ideal intention, the stated instructions, and the diverse expressions of the practice taken by the student, and in many cases this diversity is acknowledged, even encouraged by the teacher. If not, students will need to intuit how wide a gap between instruction and compliance each teacher will allow.

These gaps between the teacher's output and the students' interpretation of the practice are in fact always present both in modern postural and post-lineage teaching. But in post-lineage yoga they are a *feature* of practice evolution, rather than a *dilution* of the source of the teachings.

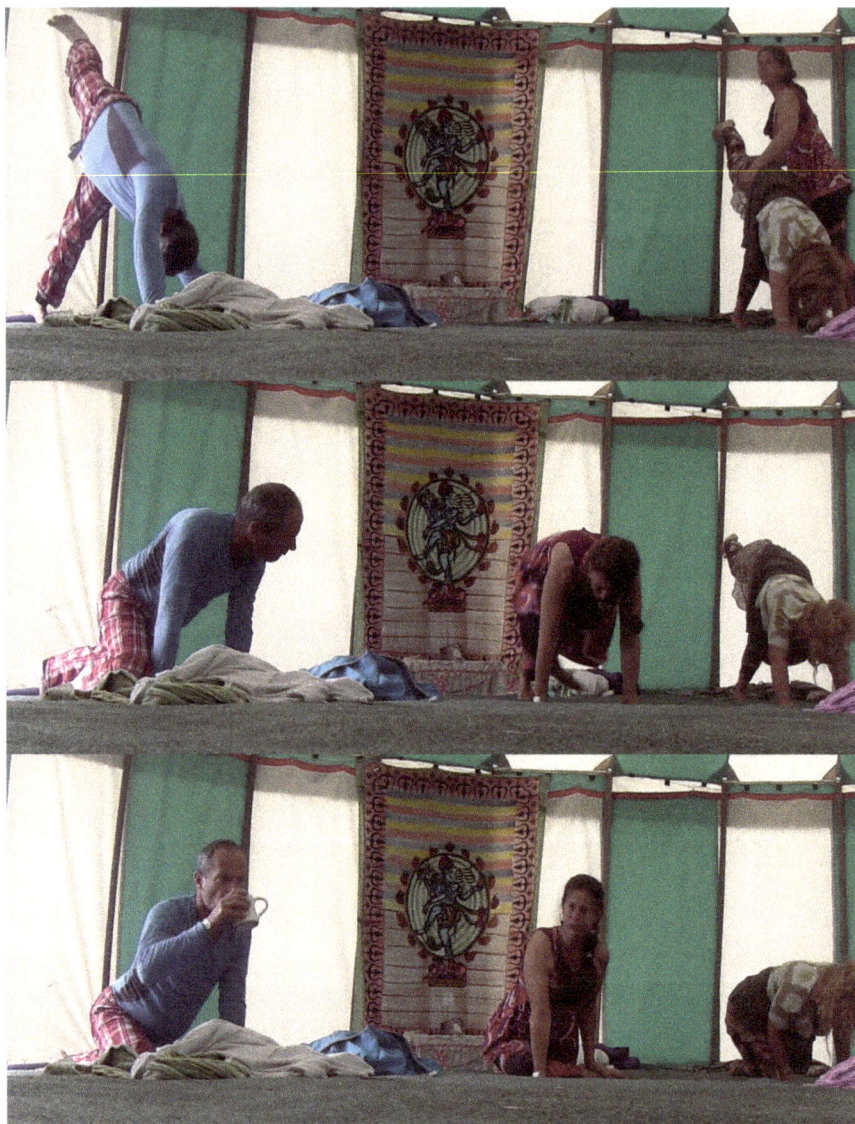

Figure 7.3
Sundara: Variations on a theme

Each practitioner's own experience contributes to the group consensus in a way that is much rarer within a set hierarchy, and consistent with the processes of personal experimentation we saw in the previous chapter. Innovation through individualisation is encouraged among students as well as teachers. Teachers accept higher levels of not just innovation, but feedback from students within sessions. And as many people take turns in the role of the teacher within the same community, this also encourages multiple and diverse iterations of the practice to be shared. The new iterations of practice that survive are those that hold true for a critical mass of engaged practitioners.

The hidden context of yoga teaching methodologies

In both modern postural and post-lineage yoga, transcendent and therapeutic intentions commonly collide (Alter 2005: 119). The transmission of contemporary yoga increasingly includes protocols of informed consent, standardised curricula, and competency tests, as in other therapeutic professions. But for many practitioners who seek spiritual transformation, the true self liberated by practice exists beyond any need for safety protocols, and the transmission that enables it is achieved by some form of divine grace. Sometimes such grace is received directly from a guru, sometimes it is experienced as an impersonal divine force, but it is always unpredictable and mysterious (Jain 2012: 20). In the modern era, group instruction as the conduit or container in which a student discovers such grace, appears incompatible with contemporary ideas of rational, informed consent. For Paolo Friere, 'knowing [...] means being an active subject who questions and transforms' (Shor 2002: 26). It is arguable that the desire to experience unpredictable encounters which remake the very self that seeks, in fact transform the apparently consenting student into an unpredictably different, previously unknowable self, and thus cannot fit any such definition of consent. And as the authority for yoga practice widens to a group of post-lineage peers, there is as yet no common discussion as to whether a group of non-enlightened humans can also be a conduit to previously unknown esoteric knowledge, becoming greater than the sum of its parts.

Whether in teaching roles that hold inherited charisma, in verbal instructions that conceal cross-cultural assumptions about physical and moral rectitude, or in physical adjustments that developed in a far more patriarchal and colonial context, riding within the content of group instruction is the transmission of diverse unseen or implicit aspects of yoga culture. Contemporary yoga is a practice of meaning-making. It is not just instructed, but variously narrated, explained and idealised.

Within post-lineage yoga, the fluidity of authority involved in distributing the role of the teacher is matched by the fluidity of identity that has been sustained, enacted and narrated through each teacher's own, individual practice. In group sessions, students are thus invited to imagine themselves as other bodies, in mythical roles, or to re-enact formative experiences, as in this dance session at Sundara:

> And I want us to get really clear with who we're with and who's in the centre. It's no longer a person. We're witnessing a dance of Mother Nature. This form, these forms are extensions of all the elements. Inside this form is all the animals, all the minerals and all the stars.
>
> (Dancing the Heart Path session, Sundara)

The most physical of instructions refer to metaphors of self-manifestation, self-liberation, and self-surrender, as in this movement session at Santosa:

> And again, let your knees find another pair of knees. And any time I invite this partner dancing, you are so welcome just to be on your own if that's what you need. If that's what your knees need.
>
> (Movement is Medicine session)

Narratives of reforming and liberating personal identity are embedded in the learnt history of many practices of yoga. The perceived moral character of a teacher is not easily separated from the practices they were responsible for innovating. When any prominent teacher is accused of unethical behaviours, well-established practices that are used both within and beyond that lineage are often reconsidered (if rarely completely abandoned) in the light of this new evidence. Some teachers and scholars are debating the origin and ongoing role of postural adjustments in all schools of yoga, in the light of accusations of sexual assault during Ashtanga Yoga classes in Mysore (Taylor 2018; Smith 2018). Others have debated the safety of all *yoganidrā* practices following evidence of abuse in the Satyananda lineage (Remski 2014a). In a statement for the **Total Yoga Nidra Network**[1] following the Satyananda investigation, Uma and her partner Nirlipta proclaim

> We are glad to be able to bring fearless independence, clarity, and critical and creative thinking to a practice that has often been hedged about with fears and dogma.
>
> (Dinsmore-Tuli and Tuli 2018c)

---

1 A learning community of post-lineage *yoganidrā* teachers co-founded by Uma Dinsmore-Tuli (Case study 3) and her husband, Nirlipta Tuli.

When a present or former devotee to a specific lineage has considered the very person of the guru to be a conduit for spiritual blessings within a practice of intimate self-discovery, and bowed year on year to the imprint of their footprints in a pair of sandals, a visceral horror is provoked by allegations and evidence of their abuse. As one Satyananda Yoga teacher put it at Santosa:

> It's the denial, the heartache, the abuse, and then the initial collusion that people go through, in order to protect themselves. [...] It's devastating.

The timing of this research coincided with increasing attention being paid in transnational yoga culture to instances of abuse by teachers at all levels of reputation, as part of a wider cultural reckoning epitomised by the #metoo movement (for examples see Carlson 2017; Rain 2018). Lineage institutions, teachers' organisations and post-lineage affinity groups alike are struggling with such issues on an unprecedented level, and responses are fast-evolving and contested. The full extent of historical or contemporary abusive behaviours by yoga teachers and gurus is thus far unclear, but probably endemic. Whether all of the most prominent yoga institutions are structurally prone to enabling it, is also unclear, but possible. There are a number of new academic research projects that aim to further explore this topic. Similar revelations within many other religious institutions, not least the Catholic Church, have provoked debates that could contain insights relevant to similar ongoing debates among yoga devotees (Orsi 2013: 4).

Understandably, the extent to which transnational yoga organisations will be able to embed restorative justice into internal processes of accountability remains to be seen. But with facilitated dialogue such as that begun at YogaCity in New York (www.yogacitynyc.com), and at the 2019 Brighton Yoga Festival panel on sexual violence, accountability and safety (at which I personally spoke), some post-lineage communities might be among those 'beloved communities' (Brosi 2012) in which healing from such abuses can begin. And it is clear that the impact of each of these spiritual crises forms a hidden landscape that underpins and continues to shape post-lineage subcultures.

The hidden processes in shared movement

Alongside the taught and led practice sessions, post-lineage events are often organised in multiple ways that increase interpersonal entrainment:

harmonising rhythms of activity and rest through shared schedules and regular communal relaxation activities such as *yoganidrā*; bringing heart and breath rates into synchrony with *bhaktiyoga*; and even sweating together in group saunas. These aspects enhance the mutuality already common to any group form of movement practice, including modern postural yoga. With a few notable exceptions, almost all contemporary yoga group sessions encourage students to move more or less in time, and that movement is synchronised to the rhythm of their breath, leading students to breathe more or less in time together. When yoga teachers additionally count breaths on behalf of participants, that entrainment to a shared rhythm of breathing becomes more marked (Schuler 2011: 97).

Many yoga teachers will encourage rising and falling patterns of effort by students, to intuitively encourage shared peak experiences, just as a DJ will use the rhythmic modulation of music to induce a similar attunement among attendees at ecstatic raves (Takahashi 2004: 154). Each post-lineage or modern postural yoga session, to borrow from acoustic terminology, might have a stronger attack, or longer sustain to its intensity, and differing rates of release into restfulness. Within the greater arc of the session may be experienced shorter modulating waves of movement sequences, just as individual chants will have their own pace and tempo within the larger *kīrtan* in *bhaktiyoga*. The intuitive practice of structuring sessions in this way is less common among teachers who focus on individualisation rather than universalised practice outcomes.

In developing the co-practice methodology for this project, I also discovered little-understood side-effects to the mimicking or repeating of physical movement. These have been a hidden factor in the teaching of yoga since the modern era, and thus group practice, began. Neurological and anthropological research suggests strong links between shared movement practices and group affinity (de Waal 2008: 287). As Maxine Sheets-Johnstone writes:

> To move among others is to be part of an interanimate world. To move in concert with others is, as indicated, to move in harmony with them. To be able to do so is to think in movement, not just one's own movement but one's own movement in conjunction with the movement of others.
>
> (Sheets-Johnstone 2017: 2)

Many movements have associations beyond the setting of a yoga session. Kundalini Yoga *kriyās* are reminiscent of held stress positions (Leach

2016: 8). Certain *āsanas* were used as postural punishment in Indian schools (Hargreaves 2017). Furthermore, simply moving side by side with others heightens empathy, which becomes especially potent in situations such as these, where other aspects of physical entrainment are also engaged, and where the shared surroundings also shape common experiences both within practice sessions and without. And although the common perception of empathy is that it is an entirely benign quality, entrainment can control, and empathy can be dangerous to either party:

> To mimic somebody or something is to be sensuously filled with that which is imitated, yielding to it, mirroring it bodily. It is, Taussig claims, a powerful way of comprehending, representing, and above all controlling the surrounding world.
>
> (Bubandt and Willerslev 2015: 17)

Independent of any intention on the part of instructor or instructed, the act of moving together, together with the attitudes that are associated with that movement, can enhance the contagion of emotion in group settings (Nummenmaa et al. 2012: 9599; Schuler 2011: 93). Thus moving, eating, and breathing together can be a source of cognitive control, whether intentional or not (Barsalou et al. 2005: 44). In shared movement, authority is leveraged not just in direct instruction, but also through entrainment, mimesis, and sympathetic magic (Bubandt and Willerslev 2015: 19).

Yoga is a practice taught and transmitted from human to human, body to body. Students learn to mirror and imitate the movement, even the breathing patterns of teachers, before they learn what these movements mean for them as individuals, and even while they are (re)creating a sustainable sense of self. Modern postural yoga is a practice built on group transmission with little understanding of the risks and rewards of group movement. Post-lineage yoga transmission democratises the authority for practice, but often deliberately intensifies the rhythmic and sustained entrainment of breath, heart-rate, trance states and even hormonal cycles in other ways. Each post-lineage event is profoundly relational, and thus in stark contrast to the intrapersonal reconciliation of self and world involved in solitary practice.

Group transmission of this kind involves mimicry, and therefore empathy, or it involves intuitive group entrainment, that transfers agency from the individual to the collective (Schuler 2011: 81). In the process, sensation, experience and intimacy is amplified. What keeps post-lineage yoga practitioners unrolling their mats alongside each other is as much the experiences of affinity that these processes of group entrainment offer, as the content of the teaching available. And so, attendees at Santosa curl up close together for a moment of shared Laughter Yoga before dinner, their heads resting on another's abdomen, and a Biodanza teacher at Sundara demonstrates finding a common rhythm with a partner, saying: 'Actually, what we're doing is revealing each other's rhythms. Dropping into one another's rhythms. It's very natural.'

The impact of charisma and interpersonal power on group instruction

In the teaching of all forms of modern and contemporary yoga we find bodies moving together, entrained and implicated in complex power relations. At post-lineage yoga events, when taking up the revolving role of the teacher, a teacher-practitioner relies on multiple sources of authority and charisma beyond their formal training and experience, and they gain further cultural status from their effective performance of the same. A teacher's value to the post-lineage subculture is calculated in the effectiveness of their taught content, their position within the community, their adaptability, and the modelling of shared ethics.

This value includes the practical skillsets, interpersonal connections and service that sustain post-lineage subculture. Subcultural status confers authenticity in the eyes of students and the consensus of the network. While some key actors in the post-lineage community are charismatic and popular teachers, others are valued for their practicality, their networking, or even their habit of challenging others productively. Organisers of events often combine many of these roles.

Each teacher's charisma is also the product of multiple sources of perceived authenticity. Authenticity can be signalled by biographical details, such as one's length of practice and depth of study, or by physical attributes such as more-than-usual abilities and unusual neurologies that suggest the supernatural, as exemplified by the impressive mobility and strength shown by Nicole (Case study 6) and Christopher (Case study 2). It can also be gained by mining the self for hagiographic and otherwise inspirational content for teaching narratives. In a Hatha Yoga session at Colourfest, the teacher's voice flowed hypnotically through a stream of consciousness narration of their own practice as students mimicked her movement, her intent and even her experience.

Find the drishti point of focus. [...] Bring equanimity into the body. [...] Finding the balance between the female and the male within the body. [...] The breath is ever-flowing. Never stop. And within that breath there is steadiness.

Just as physical attributes improved by practice are also enhanced by genetic privileges such as hypermobility or strength, so the narrative content of each session is enhanced by a teacher's storytelling ability, personal history and education. These two aspects meet in a frequently occurring disconnect between the effort the student has to put in to achieve a practice, and the performed calm of the teacher in narrating instruction. In a number of my case studies, there was a similar disconnect between the *apparent* intensity and the *narratives* participants used to explain their practice. My respondents' post-practice interpretation of challenging practices often involved emphasising significant calm, ease and joy. As Christopher said of his own apparently intense practice in Case study 2: 'Ah, that was a gentle practice today. It was just a soft practice today.'

Translated to the teaching environment this narrative strategy means that when a teacher presents or models effortlessly that which the student finds challenging, the disjunction implies expertise, with the teacher's charisma subtly signalling a level of advanced competence and experience. Conscious of this, other teachers talk of making visible their mistakes and narrating their ordinariness while teaching.

Post-lineage group teaching, and indeed much of contemporary yoga teaching, involves inspiration and aspiration, modelling and enactment, charisma and catharsis. It is a complex mix of inherited, individualised and intuited elements, and is as semiogenetic as the individual practice it relates to. It combines a repertoire of practice, some shared ethical structures and diverse techniques. But the processes of reflexive self-inquiry that are used to develop individual practice are rarely used to consider the dynamics and habits of its group teaching environments. Indeed, rarely do *any* yoga teachers consider the inherited pedagogical philosophies that govern what they teach. But just as post-lineage practitioners question the authority structures through which they inherited the practice, post-lineage teachers are at least starting to question the ways in which they pass the practice on to others.

Beyond the taught sessions of yoga, in this subculture, various talks by activists, *satsaṅga* (wisdom sharing) by religious leaders, and opportunities for *sevā* can reinforce orthodoxy, or provide much-needed hope, connection and perspective. Shared practices of *āsana*, *bhakti*, *yoganidrā* or dance, offer the mixed blessing of entrainment and emotional contagion, but are also opportunities for reconciling one's grief, whether due to a collective disillusionment with lineage, or to more individual traumas. In order to build a culture of empathy that is not devoid of ethics or agency, post-lineage yoga must continue to surround transmission with an increasingly robust culture of shared ethical norms. Teaching protocols that build healthy emotional engagement and personal agency must continue to develop in response to the increased intensity of interpersonal power issues that occur in group transmission (de Waal 2012: 135).

While the most significant transmission innovation of yoga in the modern era may well be practising as a group, both scholars and practitioners are only beginning to understand what it means for bodies to practise yoga together. Just as each individual practice is a unique iteration of post-lineage yoga, both inspired by and contributing to the subculture as a whole, so each teaching session is a unique iteration of the diverse processes that sustain and evolve the pedagogical whole. The democratisation of authority inherent to the overall endeavour is unevenly applied, and the practice cycle imperfectly translated. Yet it is the very slippage between intention and effect, and the accumulated power of diverse sources of teaching charisma, that fuel the continuation and evolution of the practice, here at least, into a coherent subculture.

8

Creating a shared repertoire

As discussed in the previous chapter, the aim of group teaching in modern postural yoga is to maintain a practice repertoire that is as close as possible to the perceived original wisdom of lineage, or the reproducible coherence of a brand. But post-lineage yoga practice diversifies much more rapidly, within subcultures that are consciously seeking its ongoing evolution. The shared repertoires of post-lineage yoga are incrementally changed by regularly incorporating new practice content. Most often, innovations or revelations that arise in individual practice are tested in group teaching environments, and those that are useful for enough students are shared by more and more teachers. Eventually, these innovations might survive to enrich enough teaching repertoires that they become part of what is seen as a common landscape of practice: a thing that is done 'by us', even if it is not a thing that 'everyone does'.

A specific post-lineage subculture, like the series of events profiled in this book, will have its own unique shared repertoire of practice. Again, not everyone will experience every practice element, but they will understand that these practices are part of the things that happen when the community comes together. Many of these elements will be familiar from diverse lineages, movement practices and other cultural sources available, although the exact mix of these varies according to the practice preferences of the people who usually attend a particular event or series of events. For example, many teaching sessions at Colourfest are influenced by the wide diversity of non-yoga movement practices also taught there, which include Contact Improvisation, and various forms of vernacular dance. In comparison, more of the practices shared at Santosa will assume a familiarity with the 'divine feminine' schools of yoga, and more of the sessions taught at Sundara will assume a familiarity with concepts of esoteric anatomy such as *nāḍīs* (energetic channels) or *cakras* (major energetic nodes).

Trends emerge over time, and some will be associated with the specific character of a particular event, while others will spread through the subculture as a whole: in the last five years, for example, all three events have held some form of ceremonial cacao ritual. Beyond this specific subculture, however, specific practices, *bhakti* chants, or particular *vinyasa* movement sequences, may have much less relevance in other communities of post-lineage yoga practice. This is unless or until they are practised and taught by *those* teacher-practitioners in *their own* shared spaces, spreading into *those* subcultures in the same way: from body to body, practice by practice.

NAVIGATING STANDARDISATION AND COMMERCIALISATION

To recap, each teacher brings a unique style to their teaching, and all of them will add new variations and innovations to the shared repertoire. But for some teachers, their own practice repertoire becomes a recognisably new form of practice. Such new content is often shared at post-lineage events, in a specific session bearing a name that recognises its newness. A yoga teacher who has spent the previous year exploring somatic approaches to movement might signal that by labelling her sessions at this year's events as 'Somatic Yoga', for example. The purpose is to test this new content with others for its coherence and transferability. The name of the session is not an attempt to brand the practice, but rather a descriptive label to help others navigate the evolving landscape of practice. Some of these new practice forms can be spontaneous and collaborative, as teachers with different approaches explore their affinities by co-teaching a session, and have to find a new and temporary label for it. The schedules for the events described in this book are filled with sessions bearing similar, descriptive labels alongside other sessions offering more widely recognised forms of yoga.

To complicate the landscape further, some of these new practice forms might be successful enough that they are formalised into a training course for other teachers. Innovating teachers may find themselves offering such training repeatedly in multiple locations, for a number of years. Increasingly, they may also package the practice and its training for digital download, such as the free yoga nidras (Dinsmore-Tuli and Tuli 2018a) and courses for sale (Dinsmore-Tuli and Tuli 2018b) at the Total Yoga Nidra Network site. If the subculture demonstrates enough demand for extensive teacher training, then the new practice form will be ratified by one of the various yoga accrediting bodies, and become a new school, rather than a new lineage.

Significantly, in the time taken to professionalise a new form of practice, a teacher's own individual practice may have evolved beyond it. The more standardised and formalised shared content becomes, the more difficult it is for it to keep pace with the teacher's ongoing development. This disconnect is increased when the content is strongly associated with the teacher's own biography. A particular practice has more shared value when it is associated with a powerful story of self-healing. *This* form of *yoganidrā* is the practice that cured one teacher's insomnia. *That bhakti* chant reflects a period of deep devotion to a specific deity. As teachers' lives evolve, such practices might decline in usefulness or importance for them personally. But these practices might continue to be the focus of their professional identity and reputation. A tension often emerges between accurately presenting one's current practice and identity, and performing a known and trusted version of themselves and their teachings. The more commercially successful a teacher's professional identity becomes, the less coherence there can be between their current individual practice and the practice that they teach to others.

Practitioners of the most visible, hyper-individual and neoliberal forms of contemporary yoga are active in their *consumption*, but disengaged from the *production* of yoga as a cultural and religious product (Jain 2014a: 76). In Andrea Jain's analysis, the affluent, white and urban learn to perform ethnically appropriated yoga practices for the price of a studio pass bought from spiritual entrepreneurs. Much of modern postural yoga thus involves packaging practices into universalised solutions, whose accompanying narratives promise wholeness, independence, health, and above all, an infinite, self-reliant abundance for the deserving (Featherstone 2010: 196; Lavrence and Lozanski 2014: 80). Many yoga teachers themselves are displeased by this trend, as typified by this satirical summary by American yoga teacher, Julian Walker:

> Now, package the image with key buzzwords from this list: intention, grace, power, heart, now, present, devotion, or freedom – and your retreat, workshop or DVD ad/print article is a wrap.
>
> (Walker 2012: 2)

Once again, there are significant differences between the transactions at the heart of commercially branded yoga as described above, and the relationships in which most post-lineage yoga subcultures evolve. Such differences extend to the creation, and above all marketing, of new subcultural content, which in post-lineage yoga develops with much more negotiation and interchange between the roles of creator and consumer. Understanding the reluctance by post-lineage yoga innovators to engage with mainstream yoga marketing tropes is key to understanding the current low visibility of post-lineage subcultures within the mainstream.

The ambivalence of post-lineage practitioners to engage with neoliberal narratives of wellbeing is more than political. It reflects a common unease with standardising and packaging any new practice, and marketing it as a universal solution to a life of easy abundance, when that message is so antithetical to the lived experiences and iterative, collaborative processes that lie at the heart of developing post-lineage practices. In this post-lineage subculture at least, there are few easy marketing stories to tell, and few simple products to package and sell. However, it is possible for commercially successful methods to be developed through post-lineage processes, but then formalise into systems of universalised content and centralised authority more consistent with established modern postural yoga transmission. New orthodoxies can arise alongside new hierarchies of authority.

Some teachers are able to create less commercial but still successful subcultural products through creative and periodic self-reinvention. Uma's published texts help to somewhat artificially separate her practices into different markets, with overlapping communities of practice: honouring the divine feminine (Dinsmore-Tuli 2013b), Celtic-inspired practices (Dinsmore-Tuli and Harrison 2015), and practices of deep relaxation (Dinsmore-Tuli and Tuli 2018c). Publishing a teacher's philosophy in book form might seem a counter-intuitive, even old-fashioned way to share embodied practices, but it provides the writer with the space needed to frame their practice with a detailed and nuanced narrative (see also Blackaby 2016; Blair 2017; Gladwell and Wender 2014). Such publications are rarely profitable in their own right. Most commonly, they modestly supplement incomes, and serve to contextualise and supplement teaching tours.

Some teachers maintain control of their shared content in ways that allow for incremental evolution by smaller affinity groups within the greater community of practice. Uma is also the co-founder of the Total

Yoga Nidra Network, which functions as a school, but also as a peer network, steadily co-evolving its field of practice with its own graduates. Each workshop, each iteration of the training manual evolves from the previous version according to ongoing feedback by associates using the material in practice. Nonetheless, in many ways a slippage still emerges, between the practice of post-lineage yoga at the point of emerging evolution, and the practice at the point of digestion into a coherent, repeatable subcultural element, whether in the form of a training manual, book, or newly named method of practice.

THE POWER OF THE TESTIMONIAL

Each form of practice will gain favour within the shared repertoire based not just on its transferable effectiveness, but also the charismatic framing and narrative coherence imbued to the practice by its originator. The most prominent, well-loved and well-connected teachers have the greatest aura of authenticity and authority, and thus the most chance of their practices entering into the common repertoire. When a narratively coherent practice meets diverse bodies, any gap in effective transmission is covered by entrainment and charisma, born in both the body and the narrative skill of the teacher. The method gains the power of a meaning-making response (Wujastyk 2011: 224). In group teaching this meaning-making is enhanced by confirmation bias (both students and teachers pay most attention to what they expect to occur); and by efficacy by association with established teachers and epistemologies (respected teachers and established 'truths' add weight when connected to new practices).

As methods grow in popularity, the semiogenetic power of the method becomes self-sustaining. Coherent forms of practice gain a reputation along with a name, enhanced by a subcultural identity that is both dependent on, and more than, the public identity of their creators. Modern postural yoga lineages are frequently named after their originators, such as Sivananda Yoga, Satyananda Yoga and Iyengar Yoga, although others, such as Ashtanga Yoga, are not. Nonetheless, early post-lineage yoga teachers such as Vanda Scaravelli and Angela Farmer, often avoided lending or refused to lend their names to any yoga school, in a conscious attempt to avoid the institutionalisation of personal charisma into newly created practice forms. Naming, standardisation, charisma, hierarchy and commercial success all correlate with wider cultural visibility, but they are often in tension with the processes of self-inquiry and individualisation necessary for post-lineage peer networks to thrive. Yet there is no clear divide to separate post-lineage from modern postural yoga here. Both exist on a spectrum.

Nonetheless, across that spectrum, in both modern postural yoga and post-lineage teaching practice, curating the narratives produced in individual practice to promote the self and one's form of yoga is common. It unconsciously adapts the hagiographic practices established by many guru lineages (Kripal 2001: 397; Venkatesan 2014: 568; Goldberg 2016a: 210), amplifies the processes of identity maintenance that are at the heart of individual practice, and follows predictable patterns. In print or in teaching, students are frequently presented with revelations that the creator of a particular practice endured some form of suffering, which was relieved in some way by the practice. These testimonies are presented within a comprehensible narrative which the student can draw on to enhance their own meaning-making response, in order to heal in similar ways.

When the teacher presenting the practice also created it, the benefits of such practices are asserted through intimate association with a personal history. By implication, to share in such practices is to learn how to embody the qualities that the teacher models in their own practice, and to overcome one's own difficult episodes with ease. Personal testimony braids together the rational and the magical in ways that repeatedly lay claim to the miracle of an everyday life lived on the edge of healing, and the edge of enchantment. Thus it is that 'in making sense of our experiences, we not only tell stories about our bodies, but we also tell stories out of and through our bodies. Here, the body is simultaneously cause, topic and instrument of whatever story is told' (Sparkes and Smith 2011: 359).

In their retelling however, these biographical testimonies begin to be abstracted and transformed, enhancing shared repertoires with an unstable form of collected and connective memory (Hoskins 2016: 349). Abstracted personal narratives, and the borrowed testimonies of others, both become part of each post-lineage teacher's repertoire. They will refer to multiple such collected histories in their teaching, overtly or implicitly re-enacting them. In essence, these are the stories 'we' tell about the practice, in the hope that 'we' also will be healed. In the process, the immediate lived experience of both students and teachers is understood, even made peace with, through that testimonial lens (Joldersma 2013: 60). A daily re-devotion to practice, and the regular performance of the outcomes of that practice, for the universal witness of the student group, enables post-lineage teacher-practitioners to tell and re-tell, frame and reframe all these testimonies of healing. The most committed students are equally invested in testimonies of healing to inspire their own self-inquiry and self-image.

The more this re-echoing and re-enactment occurs, the more the newly collective version of the narrative is refined and universalised, but also the more it is individualised to each new student enacting the practice. Post-lineage yoga repeats, but also contextualises and thus disperses the charisma associated with each practice narrative, just as it dismantles the singular systems of modern postural yoga into practice elements subject to the authority of each individual practitioner, transforming them into bespoke meaning-making for each individual repertoire.

But that process is complicated if it becomes entangled with commercial processes, because effective mass marketing fetishises heroic stories of the self, which are at odds with the cyclical processes and iterative self-development of post-lineage practice. The most effective narratives within post-lineage yoga are those that are crowd-sourced and multiple, rather than brand-approved and on-message. There must be a repertoire of diverse stories to tell, as well as diverse practices to explore. In repertoires of practice, and in the narratives that accompany them, post-lineage subcultures must intuitively maintain sufficient diversity to encourage innovation, and sufficient agreement to sustain a coherent whole.

THE SCIENCE AND FAITH SUPPORTING PRACTICE DEVELOPMENT

By now it should be clear that for post-lineage yoga teachers, citing the authority of one's own teacher or individual practice is not, on its own, sufficient rationale for a particular method or approach to practice. Post-lineage yoga draws on three types of authority when adding to shared repertoires, just as individual practitioners do with their own repertoires. One authority for practice, as demonstrated above, is the relational authority of the group. Shared experiences and shared stories both contextualise each person's access to new forms of practice. As this and previous chapters show, this process is enhanced by the visceral and emotional reality of interpersonal relationships, and the physical and narrative charisma of the teacher.

The authority of the group is, therefore, always also tested with the internal authority of the self. Individualisation and standardisation are related in complex and co-dependent ways. Each *shared* practice element is tested in the laboratory of multiple *individual* practices and experiences. As I have shown, inner wisdom is impossible to entirely separate from environments of practice, mutual entrainment and personal history. It is a combination of aspiration, experience and habitus. The teacher's own experience retains at least some influence over the lived experience of the student, no matter how temporarily those two roles may be assumed. The coherent inner self is as much the result as the authority for practice.

Lastly, we return to the external authority of the expert. Shared repertoires are enhanced by diverse sources of authoritative expertise. Recognised experts may be either internal or external to the subculture in question. A form of practice may have more authority because of its associations with a prominent post-lineage teacher, or more rarely because it is part of the repertoire of an established school or lineage. More commonly, a weight of authority is added to the shared repertoire because of connections made between its practices and some form of historical, scientific, or other scholarly research. Post-lineage yoga teachers enthusiastically engage with the outputs of scholarship not only for interest, but to add context to their practice repertoires.

As in modern postural yoga, the development of new forms of post-lineage practice frequently involves using scientific narratives as a source of borrowed authority. This is particularly common when describing the subtler results of practice, and enhances a practitioner's own confidence in the ordered safety of some very nebulous, even undefinable experiences (Remski 2015a; Alter 2005: 135). Teachers will use scientific-sounding language to describe metaphysical concepts. During Sundara's opening ceremony, one teacher described a *network* of stones all over the planet installed as an '*interface* between human world and the crystalline *grid*'. The grid's first message was an '*equation* of love'. During a Japa Yoga (chanting) session at Colourfest, even the practice of chanting *mantra* was described with a medical pun: 'We [can] have [a] heart bypass. This is a triple-mind bypass, if you're needing that.'

At some point, those teachers whose teaching narratives appeal most consistently to the authority of scientific knowledge, and who have a lay interest in biomechanics, neurology or psychology, may attempt more formal evaluations of their practice forms. The content of each practice, its usefulness for diverse bodies, and its long-term sustainability, may be studied. In reality, funding constraints and limited access to scientific research environments mean that most such practices are tested anecdotally rather than scientifically, but they still benefit from an aura of scientific accuracy and authority by including science-sounding rationales for practice choice, making reference to lay understandings and explanations of the latest research on biomechanics (Mitchell 2014), fascia (Vitalis 2016) or the polyvagal system (Sullivan et al. 2018). From Case study 1, Veronika's Reflex Yoga system is a case in point, developing as it does from lay understandings of infant development (Blomberg 2015).

As discussed in the last chapter, interpersonal entrainment and the teacher-student relationship profoundly influence the effectiveness and teaching of contemporary yoga. And yet the most common process for anecdotally evaluating new practice, consists of generalising from the teacher's narrated experience, and testing the associated new practice with sympathetic and invested students. The supportive community of practice may provide more feedback by one's peers, but further amplifies the narrative of positive benefit, for an experiment that has already lost its most critical participants (Johnson 1997: 11). If practising together involves significant empathy and entrainment, even dispersing authority from the teacher to the group cannot avoid the normative bias involved in evolving a new practice form with a sympathetic group that is invested in the outcome (Slee, Azzopardi and Grech 2012: 20).

In the end, confirmation bias and groupthink is impossible to separate from the often positive and powerful effects of entrainment, placebo, and the persuasion of a good story that is ritually told, by a teacher who truly believes in the effectiveness of the practice (Rappaport 1999: 47). What is being tested is the effectiveness of the teaching *environment*, as much as the effectiveness of a new practice form. In considering this fact, it is important to realise that this is true for most therapeutic relationships, or indeed many medical interventions (Wujastyk 2011: 223–4; Simpkin and Schwartzstein 2016). Belief, particularly in the form of embodied knowledge, is more than a form of false consciousness (Mellor and Shilling 2010: 29), and the creation of shared belief in the effectiveness of post-lineage practices is inherent to their evolution. All forms of modern and contemporary yoga teaching involve methods of interpersonal persuasion that rely on the spaces and connections *between* scientific understandings, therapeutic relationships, and faith.

CONCLUSION

Authority structures such as these that rely on intuitive peer relationships are complex and at times even incoherent (Howard 2013: 83). It is important not to overly romanticise local movements of resistance to global forces of hierarchical authority and neoliberal commercialisation. The practice of developing post-lineage yoga is much more likely to create localised alternatives than it is to challenge the dominant mainstream. Yet post-lineage yoga as a practice often does provide its practitioners with the resilience to resist and challenge authorities of all kinds, and that resilience relies on the freedom of association and innovation that its processes of vernacular authority represent (Howard 2013: 82). In contrast, the universalised forms of modern postural yoga have not enabled a safer practice or more ethical teaching relationships thus far. Standardising shared repertoires is especially problematic and endemic in those schools of practice that confuse aesthetically ideal bodies, with healthy bodies (Remski 2014c; Gilman 2014: 75).

Certainty and universalisation are the foundations of standardisation and commodification in yoga. In response, radical uncertainty in interpreting the experience of others is key to further developing the democratic, participative impulse at the core of post-lineage practice (hooks 1994: 21; Institute of Development Studies 2009: 15). As Paolo Freire memorably writes: 'Authentic liberation – the process of humanization – is not another deposit to be made in men' (1996: 60). The life-enhancing personal experiences at the heart of each new post-lineage method cannot be simply transplanted into others by rote repetition of identical practices and narratives.

To renounce universalised forms of practice and universal narratives of the benefits that result, is to model vulnerability for others, to empower individual students and to enhance the resilience of an intuitively evolving subculture. Teachers who release their role as expert creators of easily packaged practices become instead organisers of information, collators of diverse experience, and thus co-holders of a community tradition (Baistow 1994: 36). They can also retreat to a more pragmatic and less anxious self-image, no longer having to embody the perfect results of a perfect practice. Developing critical thinking in both students and teachers, developing more transparency about the sources of each teacher's knowledge, exploring more extensive teaching collaborations, and expanding peer supervision, would further deflate the lingering image of the isolated charismatic teacher who is the sole source of a complete and coherent approach to the practice of yoga. This would provide more of David Clark's 'security, significance and solidarity' for the learning communities at the heart of developing post-lineage yoga repertoires (1996: 109).

What emerges as a result is a system of peer-networked, distributed authority in which different specialists take the role of the teacher in turn, and the consensus for practice intuitively evolves in negotiation with others. This has a fitting resonance with the experience at the heart of individual post-lineage practice. The recreation of a self in real time, from multiple possible identities, is mimicked by the ongoing creation of a group identity, characterised by the shared repertoire of practice. 'We' are the people who practice these forms, who tell these stories and who share these aspirations. But just as the self is still subject to the influence of others, so even the most horizontally organised post-lineage communities are still subject to uneven relationships of power. Charisma still accrues and must be tempered or dissipated.

Charisma may be inescapable in some form. Those who hold it embody the specific values of each community within post-lineage yoga, whether they have the discipline to sustain intense physical focus, or the power to re-enchant the world through narrative. Just as the semiogenetic power of placebo can be understood and usefully harnessed for healing (Moerman and Jonas 2002: 472), so the power of charisma to provide a guiding light for the subculture can have similar positive effects.

The history of yoga shows remarkable transformations in teaching methods, from one to one tuition to mass group teaching, and from a cultural and religious practice primarily aimed at teaching men right living, detachment, and even renunciation, to a largely female-led practice for health, right relationship and self-reconciliation that aims to be inclusive to as large a population as possible. Such transformations also affect the relationships between individual practices, taught practices, and shared repertoires. Governing these relationships is the complex tripartite authority of self, expert and group, and a growing use of techniques that build agency rather than conformity among students. Complicating this picture are the flows of charisma, appeals to science, and the power of faith and **semiogenesis,** or meaning making, in the ongoing recreation of a shared practice that is as transcendent as it is therapeutic. The ongoing creation of this post-lineage subculture rests above all on a strong foundation provided by the culture and community supporting post-lineage yoga in Britain. In the following chapter I will explore in particular how rhizomatic development and a murmuration of ethical norms underpin the teaching and ongoing evolution of this remarkably innovative, individualised, yet subculturally coherent practice.

9
Culture and community

What may be most unusual about post-lineage yoga subculture as I have encountered it is the strong sense of community that supports post-lineage yoga here in the UK. The ongoing creation of new post-lineage practice is supported by an informal but vital network of peers and gatekeepers, by a shared language for ethics and experiences, and by shared experiences that take place in shared places. Such practice communities also exist in modern postural yoga, but there, hierarchical and institutional structures largely formalise the development and preservation of its shared culture. In order to thrive, post-lineage yoga has much more informal interpersonal connections to sustain.

SHARED NORMS AND A LANGUAGE FOR SHARED EXPERIENCES

The shared language of post-lineage subculture primarily serves to describe experiences or debate ethical norms. As this book has already shown, the naming of *practice forms* is uneven and imprecise, because different teachers will be working with diverse lineage sources. Different names can be given to the same practice, such as the alternate nostril breathing technique known variously as *anulomaviloma* or *nāḍiśodhana*. Other practices that share a name can have diverse features, such as the *āsana* sequence known as *sūrya namaskāra*.

It is instead in the naming and comparing of visceral and esoteric *experiences* that post-lineage yoga seeks common alignment. The typologies of post-lineage yoga borrow Tantric, Vedic, Ayurvedic, medical, Theosophical and pagan terms to describe the lived qualities of the practice. These qualities form a map that can be used to navigate the experiences of individual practice, to narrate the teaching of practice, and to categorise practices within the shared repertoire. Elements such as earth and fire, *kapha* and *pitta*, name qualities of interoceptive experience that recall object qualities of hot or cold, still or mobile. To these primal concepts are added terms that describe sensations of compression and expansion, rising and falling, as well as experiences of union and separation, cleansing and pollution, and so on.

Each of these qualities can be explored in pairs of opposites that provoke further experiences. Naming experience in this way allows practitioners to compare objective phenomena with subjective qualities: fluidity in movement is qualitatively similar to the flow of water, steadiness in posture recalls the strength of a tree trunk, and so on. Interoception thus becomes a shareable experience. We might disagree on the exact shape or name of *mālāsana* (a deep squat), but we can intuitively share the experience of pressure in the hip joints, of heaviness in the feet. Thus transmission is possible between one lived body and another (Leledaki and Brown 2009: 313), even though the language of teaching describes sensations only discovered through personal experience. In just one example, the yoga teacher leading the Women's Sauna session at Santosa leads participants in connecting to the cleansing potential of fire, through the sensation of sunlight on the skin:

> Just feel that energy of the sun. We are giving thanks to the sun. And we're connecting with that heat, with that fire. It's the heat of the fire that is the medicine in the tradition. With that heat, that fire, that helps us to cleanse. To let go of toxins but also to let go of thoughts, to let go of fears.

Much of this use of language is intuitive and metaphorical rather than explicitly typological. Indeed, the shared language of post-lineage yoga obscures a great deal of diversity in individual interpretations and experiences. Single terms contain a constellation of meanings. Once again it is the slippages between one person's experience and another's that serves to diversify the practice. The student's lived experience of the practice produces subtly different qualitative elements to that of the teacher, or the lone practitioner finds variations that for them, more reliably reproduce the qualitative effect intended in group practice.

In contrast to the intuitive use of language to share experience, shared ethical and behavioural norms are achieved through conscious debate. Just as in modern postural yoga, this references historical texts such as Patañjali's *yamas* and *niyamas,* and concepts such as *dharma* and *karma,* as described in the *Bhagavad Gītā* and elsewhere. Modern translations of these sources are diverse. There is a long history of adaptive reuse of the *Yoga Sutras* and other texts to evolve the axiologies that underpin the practice of yoga, both in India and abroad (Birch and Hargreaves 2016; Freschi and Maas 2016: 19). Alistair Shearer's translation of the *Yoga Sutras* is one of a number that are commonly found on yoga teacher training reading lists. It lists the five 'rules for living' for example, as simplicity (*śauca*), contentment (*saṃtoṣa*), purification (*tapas*), refinement (*svādhyāya*) and surrender to 'the Lord' (*īśvarapraṇidhāna*), preceded by Patañjali's five 'laws of life' as nonviolence (*ahiṃsā*), truthfulness (*satya*), integrity (*asteya*), chastity (*brahmacarya*), and nonattachment (*aparigraha*) (Shearer 2010: 107–8). Other interpretations will substitute 'sexual responsibility' for *brahmacarya* (Remski 2012: 108), or gloss *īśvarapraṇidhāna* as 'wholehearted dedication to the Divine' (Devi 2010: 170).

The various ethical norms that result from these adaptations are more than mistranslations. They apply the borrowed authority of some of the most revered texts of yoga, in order to inspire ethical ideals that sit *between* contemporary norms and pre-modern tradition. Their shifting meanings can both encourage debate and obscure difference. For example, consensus on the importance of *asteya* (integrity) is easily found. Deeper debate will reveal the diverse ways that this concept might be interpreted in practice. Once again, in modern postural yoga the ultimate authority to (re)interpret ancient texts in this way lies with the teaching hierarchy, whereas in post-lineage yoga, both peer-to-peer discussion, and a diversity of interpretations are encouraged.

Sharing experiences through qualitative language and debating ethics with peers are ongoing processes. They continually refine a subcultural consensus about the boundaries of post-lineage yoga, and the experiences at the heart of the practice. Post-lineage culture, in this wider sense that includes norms and language, as well as a repertoire of practice, evolves like the flocking or murmuration of birds (Goodenough et al. 2017). The flock finds a consensus intention, but this is continually changing, a product of a process in which each individual finds their own route forward, while simultaneously ensuring that they do not stray too close to other members, nor too far from the group as a whole. The shared culture that results is an aggregate of the whole, flowing together. Multiple evolving, self-reconciling individuals take turns to step into the role of leading change just as members of some flocks of birds will take turns taking point. Sometimes, thus, the subculture moves like a murmuration and other times like a migration flight (Voelkl and Fritz 2017), but any post-lineage subculture in which the right to determine the pace or direction of change became permanently assigned, would cease to be *post*-lineage at all.

POST-LINEAGE PRACTITIONERS AS A 'COMMUNITY OF PRACTICE'

A post-lineage community is sustained by members who have different and evolving levels of engagement with the subculture. At the centre are a few key figures, who are connected not just to many other members, but also to many sources of cultural inspiration. For the community profiled in this book, this includes other, overlapping communities, such as Shakti Dance teachers, *kīrtan* musicians, and facilitators of Contact Improvisation. Although events are intended to be accessible to all, most first-time attendees discover these events by word of mouth. They will need to know the people that know that an event is happening, and they will still need the time and resources to attend. Access to the subculture is thus filtered through multiple gatekeepers, including those who organise events, those who decide who will teach there, and the owners of the land itself. There are schedules and roles to agree, tickets to buy and expenses to be paid. Roles and positions are fluid. A person who organises one event may volunteer at another. A teacher on the schedule of one event may run the kitchen on a different occasion. Each post-lineage event has a different configuration of gatekeepers, key figures, and teachers, and thus the authority to determine post-lineage yoga practice is also fluid, held not by a hierarchy, but by key roles within a coherent process.

Post-lineage yoga forms what Etienne Wenger first called 'communities of practice' (Wenger 1999: 78). The structure of a community of practice shapes its social relations, but is also the output of those same relationships (Sewell 1992: 27). A community of practice, according to Wenger, shares a set of *cultural resources, tasks* and *norms*. A *post-lineage* community of practice shares a repertoire of yoga practice, but also a repertoire of ways to share that practice, and a repertoire of shared stories about the community itself. Each event involves the repetition of evolving narratives about the history and future of particular events, as immortalised on the Santosa website:

> As we gear up for the most fabulous Santosa Yoga and Bhakti camp ever, I felt some of you might be interested to know the inside story of how this heart-warming yoga and *bhakti* event came to be.
>
> (Dinsmore-Tuli 2013a)

Each event is more than an opportunity to explore a shared cultural *repertoire*, however. The *sevā* or service that enables the event to take place is both a communally negotiated shared *task*, and a shared *norm*: participation of some kind is expected and rewarded (Wenger 1999: 78). *Sevā* strengthens the interpersonal relationships that sustain the community of practice. Even a well-established event could vanish from one season to the next, if the handful of people in its organising group lose the capacity or will to continue.

> We do live fairly spontaneously I would say. And so, for us committing to doing a camp once a year and saying 'Yes that's what we're going to do' is quite challenging for us.
>
> (Tanya, speaking as co-organiser of Sundara)

In 2019, the organisers of Colourfest decided to take a sabbatical year, and the event left a gap in the calendar of post-lineage events. If Robbie and Rowan decide not to return after a second year, the community of practice will either find another event to attend in early summer, or start a new festival entirely.

Overall, however, the subculture continues to thrive because the people at its heart understand that the core activity of these events is *the making and maintenance of relationships through shared practices*. While modern postural yoga is characterised by its individualism (Newcombe 2011: 218; Urban 2000: 296), they are filled with moments of intimate communal practice: the dance sessions, the *kīrtans*, the *yoganidrās* and the *pūjās*. As Rowan co-organiser of Colourfest, says:

> The yoga element is the solitary, you're a solitary person on the mat by yourself. But there is another avenue for learning which is through contact and through interaction.

It is those communal activities, rather than the more popular *āsana* workshops, that draw the largest proportion of the subculture's most dedicated members. Cooperative, performative, and improvisational activities at all these post-lineage events, strengthen the affinity of a collective whose agency is distributed among its key members (Da'oud 1997: 74–5) supporting the flocking of shared cultural evolution described above.

Flocking, whether by birds in flight, fish in shoals or any number of other examples of similar emergent behaviour, always depends on shared physical presence and entrainment (Schuler 2011: 81). Flocking is an

activity done with the body: an instinctive, moment to moment evalua-
tion of the comfort and discomfort of proximity and distance, of choice
and mimicry, of safety and innovation, between the group and the individual (Goodenough et al. 2017: 14). The most sustainable and coherent
post-lineage communities of practice devote considerable resources to
significant shared physicality and emplacement.

POST-LINEAGE TEACHING AS RHIZOMATIC LEARNING

Teachers of modern postural yoga tend to employ a very different metaphor to a flock of birds when describing the evolution of practice. The
most common is that of yoga as a tree, whose branches represent the
diverse schools, all dependent on the wisdom of the gurus at its ancient
roots (see for example YogaDork 2014). These are apt metaphors for the
development of pre-modern yoga into modern postural yoga, especially
with reference to the Mysore Palace era as described by Mark Singleton
(2010). The narratives of the most dominant schools of modern postural
yoga still trace their roots back to Krishnamacharya as a common ancestor
in the early-twentieth-century developments of the Mysore Palace, and
are dependent on the enduring reputation of each teacher or guru that
links them to that point. But my use of the term post-lineage is predicated
on the realisation that much of contemporary yoga practice not only
evolves like a murmuration, but is also governed by a *rhizomatic* authority
structure, by which I mean a learning community that is diverse, hetero-
geneous, and multiply connective.

The concept of rhizomatic learning is not new. As Lionel and Le Grange
explain, theories of learning that make use of tree-based metaphors
create not diversity, but 'pseudomultiplicities' (Lionel and Le Grange 2011:
746). These support variation *only* when it is both dependent on and subordinate to a central source. In contrast rhizomatic learning structures
disrupt orderly transmission and fixed hierarchies of authority. Just as
post-lineage instruction includes common appeals to the 'heart as inner
teacher' in each student, so the subculture as a whole is theoretically
dependent on the authority of every teacher at the centre of a class. Yet
in reality their authority here depends on their networked connection to
the rest of the subculture, and their ability to hold a participative space
for the learning community of each class. Just as the 'inner teacher' in
practice emerges as a consensus among multiple voices of the self, so each
post-lineage yoga teacher returns again and again to the shared repertoire

as the source of their evolving teachings. This is a significant evolution from the ideal of the teacher who draws only from the authority of their own teacher, in a generational hierarchy reaching back to a single, unifying lineage source for authority.

Rhizomatic learning structures often arise intuitively, and their purpose is to propagate both diversity and resilience through webs of knowledge that connect practitioners in non-hierarchical and evolving ways. As I have shown, many post-lineage communities of practice begin with those who have weathered a scandal of some kind in the lineage that trained them. This often damages their trust in the organisation that governs their ongoing practice development. Even though they are joined by those with more cordial relationships to lineage, in post-lineage yoga it is always rhizomatic communities, not individual teachers and their branching lines of followers, that produce the shared repertoire of practice (Neitz 2013: 60).

Michel Bauwens uses a more digital metaphor for similar learning structures, in an online manifesto for 'peer to peer' spirituality. As he writes:

> What is important here is not to see spiritual achievements like 'enlightenment' as transcendent qualities that trump all others and infer an unchallengeable authority on one person, but rather as particular skills that deserve respect [...] That means *no more gurus, just skilful teachers with a particular job to do.*
>
> (Bauwens 2014, emphasis added)

Post-lineage communities of practice also take their inspiration from the *saṃgha*s and ashrams that quietly supported each charismatic teacher or guru. Even within post-lineage yoga communities, some gurus who have died act as talismans of authenticity and slipped signifiers for authority. Around their memories smaller affinity groups of practitioners can maintain the illusion of shared adherence to a perfect, external authority while in fact evolving pragmatic systems of decision-making between them, which are consistent with the wider post-lineage community of practice. In fact, it may be that similar rhizomatic communities have played a much larger role in the evolution of yoga than guru hagiographies suggest (Kripal 2001: 397). Patterns of rhizomatic learning are hard to distinguish without a significant investment in ethnographic study.

Rhizomatic development is diverse, often chaotic, but profoundly resilient, as it is never dependent on a single person, group, brand or lineage for survival (Lionel and Le Grange 2011: 746). In post-lineage yoga, each teacher, each affinity group of devotees or practitioners, holds their own roots, while also recognising that they are stronger by association with many others. Nonetheless, this metaphor conceals a more complex reality. For the patterns of association, interdependence, and growth in a rhizomatic authority structure are never free from interpersonal power dynamics. As discussed earlier in this book, the rhizomatic learning communities of post-lineage yoga are strongly influenced by interpersonal affinity. The shared goal of teachers at these events is an exchange of useful practices between a trusted circle of experts, taking the role of the teacher in turn. But the events also depend on visceral contact and connections between people moving together, struggling together, liking and loving each other. Within shared ecologies, and intimate physical connections, the relationships that result are diversely intimate, and interpersonal conflict inevitably arises (Wenger 1999: 77).

Expanding on those Patanjalian ideals described above, the ethical norms of post-lineage yoga communities include: fairness to others, personal equanimity, and honesty. These norms can be difficult to reconcile when publicly discussing private conflicts (Ridout 2008: 18). Of the dispute that led to John and Tanya leaving Santosa, Uma carefully says:

> They brought their whole ex-rave festival vibe. Sorted it out. [...] and then needed to go on and do their own thing.

John and Tanya in turn emphasise acceptance when talking about the end of their involvement in Santosa, saying:

> I'm one of those people that will brush myself off and start again.
>
> (Tanya)

> I'm quite happy to walk away because I know we could always recreate what we did anyway.
>
> (John)

Like many rhizomatic communities of practice, this subculture involves not just friendly collaboration, but also discretely passionate romances, hidden disputes, injuries, illness and quietly broken friendships. The effects of these also shape post-lineage repertoires of practice. New liaisons can spark newly inspired collaborations. When organisers discover irreconcilable differences, break away groups often start new events.

Post-lineage yoga events are both ritualised and social gatherings, and they are complex experiences: meaningful and deeply felt, idealistic and carnal (Olaveson 2004: 88).

POST-LINEAGE PLACES AS SACRED SPACES

Post-lineage transmission, then, travels not just through individual and shared practice, but also through the messiness and enduring inequality of human relations (Spivak 2008: 78). It is also held in space: emplaced within the various spaces of its group events (Tweed 2006: 97). It is, like most contemporary religious subcultures, not only drawing from multiple and diverse roots, but both 'dwelling' and 'crossing' (Tweed 2006: 74). The many ways in which post-lineage practice honours the land on which it meets, the rhythms that govern its days, and the creatures that share its spaces, signify a commitment to the places of practice that is more than practical: it is an ethical, even religious endeavour. The summer events are echoed by many smaller ones across the country, marking the turning of the year in a series of events, as each teacher leads winter retreats and seasonal workshops, and each *bhakti* musician holds gatherings around holy days and holidays.

At the summer events themselves, post-lineage teaching and practice make a virtue of contingency and adaptiveness. While established schools and brands of yoga are more likely to teach predictable practices in contained spaces, in the post-lineage environment a teacher's social capital is determined by their responsiveness to circumstance and place. Event participants are also ambulant beings. They walk to connect, weaving the event together in unpredictable moments of meeting and greeting on the land, forming and repairing affinitive networks with each moment of connection, like the indigenous communities described by Lye Tuck-Po (2008: 24). Bodies here are always meeting: either exchanging words and smiles with other people, or meeting the land itself with every step. Walking feet take the paths that the land offers to them, but also change the ground beneath them. Paths become wider and firmer with use. Dance floors are created by dancing feet. Every participant is involved in the conception, construction and maintenance of space (Knott 2009: 156; Tweed 2006: 82).

Interpersonal networks of connection include other creatures, plants, and even the land itself. Human and other than human beings interact with each other in many ways (Ingold 2016: 64), and the subculture recognises many of those non-human beings as in some way conscious, and all of them as worthy of respect (Harvey 2006: 27). The aim of post-lineage practice can be understood as the reconciliation of the internal and external sacred living landscape as one, but also in community with other reconciled beings. As one teacher put it, in an Earth Dance session at Colourfest:

> Your centre is connected to the cosmos. [...] And then everything else can happen around this very calm, connected centre.

Each event is itself a coherent instance of ritualised, enacted and emplaced practice (Grimes 1995: 228). It entails mutual exchanges that transform the subcultural resources that it shares, in an unending process with no true origin point.

Those at the heart of the subculture may retain a connectedness to specific lineages and traditions, but their rootedness is also rhizomatic to each other, and emplaced, in the land (Pye 2013: 249). One teacher at one event repeated a phrase from a teacher of their own: 'It's just an excuse to all be in the same room together'. But in this case, that room is a field, meadow, country park or copse that also takes an active part in the meeting.

While transnational yoga continues to debate the tension of authority and ownership between ideas of 'India' and 'the West' (Long 2014: 126; Beckerlegge 2011: 41; Jain 2014b: 429), post-lineage subculture here both complicates and partly reconciles that division, because it is in the process of developing a form of practice, of transmission, and therefore of authority, that is uniquely emplaced. It adapts dawn fire rituals to frosty conditions at the Beltane Bhakti Gathering. It flows osmotically through canvas walls in transient spaces. This is a form of yogic cultural capital based not in the length of your lineage, but in one's commitment to ongoing exploration, and in one's ability to negotiate with others, be they land or people.

POST-LINEAGE YOGA AS A RADICAL ACTIVITY

As I have explained, post-lineage yoga practice is not inherently a political activity. However, the individual practice of post-lineage yoga and other forms of mindful movement and stillness can be a natural support for politically radical activities and identities (Rowe 2015; Schnabele 2013: 148). The practice of post-lineage yoga is an incrementally transformative activity. Furthermore, post-lineage events are zones of proximal development and liminality, in which the support of the group enables the evolution of each individual (Junker 2013: 168), and the flocking of cultural norms allows the subculture to share an identity distinct from that of commercial yoga brands or traditional schools of modern postural practice.

Post-lineage practice here is part of both emplaced and trans-locative transformations of modern postural yoga. It is connected to a local, particularly countercultural heritage. But it is equally in an uncomfortable dialogue with postcolonial struggles and diverse transnational responses to late stage, neoliberal capitalism. Modern postural yoga continues to trade on the writing of such diverse radical cultural activists as Gandhi, Thoreau, Yeats and Crowley (Godrej 2012: 437–8; Harding 2006: 10; Urban 2004: 724), but often decontextualises citations in ways that support cultural norms (Jain 2014a: 46). Key teachers and texts within post-lineage yoga continue to take similar inspiration in developing countercultural inspiration from historical figures. In *The Celtic School of Yoga* a 'hidden lineage' of 'radical' Anglo-Celtic practitioners and poets is described, inspired both by yoga and each other:

> *Yogis* [male practitioners] from this hidden lineage include W. B. Yeats and his boyhood hero, Henry David Thoreau, writer, eco-activist and advocate of civil disobedience. *Yoginis* [female practitioners] include the Irish educator and campaigner for Indian independence and women's rights, Sister Nivedita, and writer and philosopher Annie Besant.
> (Dinsmore-Tuli and Harrison 2015: 98, italics in the original)

But in Britain at least, post-lineage subculture is part of what Robert Orsi calls 'a great refusal', in this case referencing that heritage as a foundation for rejecting both patriarchal and dominant lineage structures, commercialised modern postural yoga, and indeed, neoliberalism in general (2012: 154). Here the personal and the political are consciously explored. Post-lineage yoga here also inherits some of its more eclectic practice influences from British countercultural experimentations of the sixties and seventies, including therapeutic practices based on core shamanism (Harvey 2006: 142) and Tantric sex-magic (Urban 2004). While 'for Crowley and his students, sexual magic offered a powerful source of transgression' (Urban 2004: 669), shamanic, sensual and magical practices have since been domesticated as processes of personal development (Urban 2000: 280). Post-lineage yoga subculture deliberately transgresses contemporary neoliberal norms instead through the variously applied ethics of non-consumption and non-transactionality, as well as actions in solidarity with migrants and other vulnerable groups.

Furthermore, original countercultural movements survive in Britain that some scholars have declared finished, including that of Osho (Urban 2000: 291). Devotees from the UK Osho Leela Centre hosted the 2016 Beltane Bhakti Gathering, and led a workshop at Colourfest in 2016 on the theme of 'Reclaim Your Power'. Osho Leela is also one of the few spaces outside of the Art of Living community that is exploring substance-free yoga-rave hybrids (Jacobs 2017; Jacobs and Wildcroft 2017) at their Puravida Wild Weekender events. And diverse forms of dynamic meditation and ecstatic movement are no longer 'uniquely Rajneeshian' (Urban 2000: 290), if they ever were, and are in fact a common feature of post-lineage yoga events here. There are sessions labelled 'Dance into connection' and 'Bhajans and medicine songs' (as at Colourfest in 2016), 'Bhaktiyoga Movement' and 'Dance Mandala' (as at Santosa in 2016), and 'Drumming for Deep Listening Meditation' and 'Yoga and Shamanic Meditation' (as at Sundara in 2016). Finally, in ritual practice, especially an emphasis on the care of *mūrtis*, Santosa in particular recalls not just Hindu practice, but very similar altar maintenance within the nearby Glastonbury goddess worship community (Whitehead 2008: 182).

Whether casual participants are conscious of it or not, this counter-cultural heritage is part of the fertile soil of post-lineage yoga in Britain, and its places and people continue to fertilise its growth. They are part of providing the means and boundaries for change, many of the methods practitioners adopt, and some of the shared language that the subculture speaks (Shor 2002: 35). However, it is not obvious whether attendance at post-lineage events encourages the more disparate pool of *casual attendees* to live a significantly more reflective, collectivist, or activist life. Indeed, some commentaries on the 'therapeutic turn' would strongly suggest the contrary (Apperley, Jacobs and Jones 2014: 727). There is an evident gap between the intentions of casual attendees and the flocking norms of committed practitioners. Yet teaching post-lineage yoga involves the development of personal agency, as well as self-awareness. In some teaching sessions, participant bodies are encouraged to be self-aware, and self-accepting, but also to build strength, resistance and transformative power, as in the Kundalini Yoga session led by Tanya (Case study 5) at Sundara, in which she says: 'Try not to move a muscle. We are building nerves of steel'.

Many regular participants experience these events as a space of sanctuary and nourishment, set against the significant stressors for anxiety and exhaustion found in wider culture. The use of wellbeing practices is a problematic response to socio-politically elevated levels of anxiety and a 'beleaguered self', because it substitutes personal adaptation for political change (Apperley 2014: 738). But for contemporary yoga teachers, one significant source of stress is the competitive prosperity doctrines that structure the market for teaching contemporary yoga, as described early in its development by Paul Heelas (1993: 107), and discussed by many yoga commentators, including teacher Kimberley Johnson (2011). Yoga teaching can demand a significant investment of emotional labour into the student body, and its providers are, in the majority, women. The nature of the emotional labour involved is professional and therapeutic in nature (Wharton 2009: 152), without any significant structures for peer or managerial support. Yoga teachers and allied independent therapeutic professionals are often part of the precariat of the emotional labour force (Savage et al. 2013: 230; Standing 2011: 3).

Advice available to struggling yoga teachers in a transnational, freelance market is exemplified by this affirmation-heavy and exhausting advice found in a blog post of 'steps to success for new yoga teachers' from 2015:

> Take one small action every day that moves you closer to manifesting your intention. Have the courage to say yes. [...] Unless you're legitimately underqualified, say yes anyway. Maybe you'll get a desperate last-minute call to sub a world-famous yoga teacher's class of 100-plus students. This is the universe offering you the motivation to tap into your deepest potential to fill some big shoes. Affirm yourself. Repeat after me: I am calm. I am confident. I am worthy. I am wise. [...] Add affirmations to squelch your own limiting thoughts, and repeat them daily.
>
> (Levasseur 2015)

For the committed community of my research, post-lineage community events are spaces of temporary autonomy and solidarity deliberately removed from such pressures. For many they are also places in which they can build resistance and resilience, and model alternative and intentional structures of community and exchange. Small but significant numbers of long-term attendees share stories of coming to post-lineage events as a gateway activity to substantial personal life changes. These often include giving up mainstream employment or moving into an alternative community.

Often, these changes are consistent with a longer history of countercultural engagement. There are activists here who came of age camping out at nuclear installations, and former members of eco-housing co-operatives. They join those who raised families at less-than-legal encampments such as Tipi Valley, and more transient figures who survived governmental repression of the New Age traveller lifestyle, like the activist in Calais that Ian from the One Spirit Ashram Kitchen describes below: 'She's hardcore. And she's a traveller. That's what her history is, living on the road, and living as a traveller or on sites all her life in Holland or all about the place.'

They are joined by, and encourage solidarity with, more recent movements for protest and socio-political change, in the form of anti-fracking protesters, refugee crisis workers, and campaigners against climate change and the new runway at Heathrow airport. The numbers of those engaged in the most unlawful and health-endangering of these activities may be small. But the subculture as a whole is greatly supportive of both anti-establishment politics and non-violent direct activism.

At post-lineage events, the attempt to recruit participants to personal political action is made through multiple overt and indirect methods. At the Beltane Bhakti Gathering, all attendees were encouraged to experiment with cold showers and smaller food portions, as a way to explore the event's theme of 'consuming less and contributing more'. Speakers from social justice campaigns including Compassionate Revolution (a forerunner to Extinction Rebellion) were a daily feature at Sundara. On a more pragmatic level, at Santosa's morning meetings new arrivals were taught how to squat and use a compost toilet. At all the events, campaigning messages are deliberately delivered in spaces when as many attendees as possible are present, such as in chai shops, or before highly anticipated activities.

More casual attendees are often as content to embrace organic, vegan, collectively produced food for a week, as they are to exchange it for the convenience of the supermarket as soon as they leave. Post-lineage events provide an immersion into entrainment, and thus empathy, and an introduction to post-lineage norms and behaviours which are often at odds with contemporary society. It provides access to conversations with established activists, and the opportunity to engage in low-risk, entry-level political actions. While the heart of the community maintains often surprisingly revolutionary social and political ideals, it is less clear whether the skills and repertoires which are most often taught at post-lineage events, effectively train more casual participants in a way that empowers *political* discernment, or *political* enactment.

CONCLUSION

That supportive local network that contributes to the strong sense of community that holds and supports post-lineage yoga here in the UK may be unique. It functions in many ways to support the continuing evolution of both teaching and subcultural transmission. The peer networks involved are both coherent and resilient, and support a range of levels of engagement by participants, while supporting a large core of committed community members. Post-lineage events serve as both an introduction to the subculture and vital ongoing support for key members. Although cultural capital is affected by personal charisma, and interpersonal conflict occurs, these have positive benefits also, in the form of transformational power for transmission and subcultural propagation respectively. This community of practice is supported by a common language for experience, and for ethical norms, which enhance transmission and partially counteract the solipsistic tendencies inherent in this strongly interoceptive practice.

The subculture is informed by its history, and by the shared places of its events, which also shape both practice and transmission in significant ways. That history includes the continuance of a British counterculture that many researchers have declared defunct. How far post-lineage yoga as a practice, set of teachings, and subculture, can provide a more widespread entry into new forms of activism, and new forms of communal and ethical living, remains to be seen. For post-lineage yoga to develop a practice that promotes ever more equitable inter-relationship, it would need to embrace even more diversity (Foldy 2004: 533), and further develop practices that shift each person's identity from dominant mainstream norms to a greater alignment with marginalised populations (hooks 1989: 21). This would mean including more challenging postcolonial and non-neurotypical narratives, bodies and identities, (Gaard 2001: 19) and narratives that include more than just human perspectives. It implies ever remembering that the land on which it thrives is not a silent, nurturing partner to its endeavours, but a fully realised agent and actor (Bennett 2002: 69). It means continuing to develop practices that 'build nerves of steel' and train bodies for active, non-violent resistance, but also the exploration of yoga practices that can hold and heal more significant numbers of aging, grieving, traumatised and disabled bodies, all while providing its core constituency with vital experiences of nourishment and sanctuary (Steinberg and Shildrick 2015: 16).

10
Conclusion: a global movement

THE EMERGENCE OF THE TERM 'POST-LINEAGE YOGA'

At the start of this research, my aim was to provide a vivid portrait of a living subcultural practice that was largely invisible, and to centre an investigation into contemporary yoga on those perhaps most invested in its continuing transmission: yoga teacher-practitioners. In the process, I created new research tools, and uncovered a vibrant, diverse, and locally embedded, vernacular religious form. But I also uncovered significant and coherent activities and norms that support the development of that subculture. It has become clear that those activities and norms are much more widespread than I initially suspected.

Both the subculture described here, and the processes that determine its ongoing creation, are herein given a new label: post-lineage yoga. That label, which took over a year to properly define, generates new analyses of contemporary yoga by focusing attention on the interpersonal, and on the actual mechanisms of developing, sharing and teaching yoga that have been largely absent from previous research. The process of defining post-lineage yoga was dependent on developing and testing the new methodology that allows post-lineage processes to become visible. It is my hope that the specific conclusions and the methods described in this book inspire other researchers to join me in re-evaluating the history of teaching yoga within vernacular communities of practice.

My research clearly shows how in a *post-lineage* yoga subculture, communal experiences and shared accounts of individualised experience serve together to expand and confirm each person's affordances to new ways of practice, and new ways of living, as part of peer networks of shared knowledge generation. It is that network of highly invested peers, and the shared roots and shared nourishment that they maintain, that prevents dominant hierarchies from arising. While we can expect similar processes of peer exchange to be present to an extent in both lineage and brand communities, in those communities the flows of horizontal transmission are far more subordinate to the vertical authority of institutional hierarchy.

In lineages such as Sivananda Yoga, the set practice sequences of the guru maintain their status as pristine originals, and extensive adaptation is frowned upon. Teaching Bikram Yoga and some aspects of Satyananda Yoga involves the repetition of set scripts to frame a pre-set practice. And the majority of lineages and brands remain highly suspicious of any new content that comes from outside of their specific institution. A teacher's identity as, for example, an Iyengar Yoga teacher is constrained by the avoidance of practice content considered to be foreign to the Iyengar system, *even if it is created by another well-recognised yoga school or lineage.* No matter how diverse, each modern postural yoga repertoire is consistent with a single identity consistent with the school and founder.

Democratically developing content, and sharing it with others regardless of affiliation, is definitional of post-lineage yoga. Thus, while individual teachers, organisations, and events might be positioned on a continuum of modern postural to post-lineage yoga activities, its two poles are defined by the acceptability at one end of creating and adopting new practice content, and explicit or implicit protocols disallowing this at the other. And as I showed through the practice structure of audit, remedy, *innovate* and savour, innovation at the level of the individual practitioner is a key element of everyday post-lineage practice.

It is therefore significant that the label 'post-lineage yoga' is already being discussed, debated, and used to apply to subcultures outside of my research by practitioners themselves: first used publicly by J. Brown (2017a, 2017b), discussed with David Lipsius of Yoga Alliance (Lipsius and Wildcroft 2018) and referenced by Peter Blackaby (2018), among many others, including a number of those included as case studies in this book. Uma's (Case study 3) own Yoga Nidra Network now describes itself as 'proudly post-lineage'. This term has much to offer individual practitioners in understanding their own processes of practice and teaching. As its findings become more well-known, this term is also increasingly provoking more communal debates, a number of which I have been invited to help facilitate. Such group discussions are enabling a shared recognition by post-lineage subcultures of the activities that sustain them. In the process, my positionality as researcher, consultant, and facilitator becomes ever more complex to navigate. I continue to see my role as one of service: to hold up a mirror to the communities of post-lineage yoga, that they might see themselves more clearly, but not to dictate what they do in response to that clarity.

Personal communications with well-known writers on contemporary yoga, such as Carol Horton (2018), and Jacqueline Hargreaves (2018), as well as references in more recently published texts (Remski 2019: 282), suggest that the term 'post-lineage yoga' is also an extremely useful one to think with for scholars and other commentators in Yoga Studies. With this term, we are better able to understand an unevenly applied but increasingly conscious development in the transmission of yoga practice. The co-practice method is also a particularly fruitful way to study practices that are both movement repertoires, and sites of meaning-making. It would enhance any interdisciplinary study comparing the kinaesthetic phenomenology of movement, familiar from dance studies, and the somaesthetic phenomenology of stillness, familiar from studies of religion. The notation method, and the broader concepts of methodology as experiment, and methodological *sevā* or service, are also useful concepts to contribute to the study of religion more broadly. By engaging with the conceptual framework of post-lineage yoga, it is my hope that both scholars and practitioners will understand the interpersonal relationships that support this deeply interoceptive practice, and in the process better define, and better sustain, contemporary yoga practice.

Vernacular subcultures such as those practising post-lineage yoga are an understudied phenomenon (Bender 2012: 281; Primiano 1995: 38). The scope of this research, as a doctoral project with a single researcher, could not contain a full analysis of post-lineage yoga as a widespread evolution in the transmission of yoga practice. At every stage of the research project however, wider implications of the data under consideration became clear. This book makes a significant academic contribution: to ongoing debates about the embodied positionality of the researcher; to the study of vernacular and lived religious practice, and to what Tweed describes as 'the role of personal agency in the kinetics of religious dwelling and crossing' (2006: 176). While Aristotelian definitions of the esoteric are of those practices that necessitate oral transmission and presence (Encyclopædia Britannica 2016), much more work remains to uncover the mechanisms, risks and rewards of the kind of in person, embodied and esoteric transmission that post-lineage yoga practice exemplifies.

A COMMON PROCESS PRODUCING UNIQUELY EMPLACED SUBCULTURES

The post-lineage community profiled in this book is therefore only one such uniquely evolving subculture. Its shifting network comprises a community of practice that sustains its members against the anxieties and injuries of both daily life, and the pressure and isolation of teaching yoga in more mainstream environments. In coming together, this subculture is further engaged in communal and overtly religious activities at odds with descriptions of transnational yoga as a largely secular, individualised, and casual affair. Such activities include a particular focus on *bhakti* and *sevā* as acts of devotion and service that are also acts of community and social justice. The events themselves become unique iterations of shared practice, and shared liminality. While this is a community that accepts diverse levels of engagement, those that organise, maintain, and teach at these events form a core community that can outnumber more casual involvement. They are highly invested in the subculture, with a multiply connected or rhizomatic structure of interrelations.

As a vernacular practice however, post-lineage yoga is in part defined by its defiance of labels. Its more reflexive members are actively engaged in reassessing a number of key concepts of modern postural yoga: from *ahiṃsā* to alignment, from *sevā* to the role of the teacher. Each individual practice is thus a unique iteration of post-lineage yoga. Each practitioner negotiates an individualised axiology and ontology. Each person encountered in my research negotiates a unique journey of collaboration and individual expression, both conforming to and questioning the teachings that they receive directly, modern postural yoga norms, and contemporary society. Each teacher has a recognisable, individual style, even when they collaborate with other teachers. Each organiser has their own priorities, and co-creates a uniquely recognisable event within the summer schedule. Beyond the three events and key figures of this research are many others. The resulting inter-relationship between social and political radicalism, teaching style, and questioning lineage is complex and individual. The members of the core community are far more self-aware than the average contemporary yoga practitioner described in previous scholarship. But regardless of their level of investment each practitioner is also part of a significant, coherent, previously unidentified subculture. Its ethics, teaching protocols and practices are ever evolving, and some individuals are more active in that evolution than others, but the subculture negotiates these trends collectively, and largely democratically.

In the specific environments of my research, that subculture is part of a countercultural heritage that a number of scholars with a North American focus in particular, have declared extinct (Urban 2000: 291; Jain 2014a: 21).

Nonetheless, while there are many shared subcultural reference points described in this book, any typologies of a post-lineage practice repertoire will always be incomplete, given how rapidly and diversely each post-lineage subculture evolves. For this research project, it was vital instead to determine the process of mapping and sharing that repertoire that happens during individual and group practice. The practice cycle begins in auditing the self, moves to mining the existing repertoire for remedies, on to innovating new practice elements, and savouring the results of that practice. It can be described independently from the practice repertoire, and is thus likely to be of interest to other researchers of yoga and similar practices.

Adapting from Michel de Certeau's understanding of mysticism, dedicated post-lineage practitioners are seeking: a place in which to move; a different conception of subjective identity; and a new repertoire of movement (Blevins 2008: 39). The practice cycle therefore produces a creative tension found in many historical and contemporary forms of yoga: between introspective reception, and intentional expression, with the aim of evolving some new experience of the self. In post-lineage yoga shared practice also exists in productive tension with individualised practice, as both are in conversation, and governed by the practice cycle. The porousness between self and group practice is mirrored in the attempted reconciliation between internal selfhood and external ecology by each practitioner.

The use of practices of stillness and movement to evolve identity in this way is not unique to the yoga described here. But it is promoted by post-lineage yoga's emphasis on iterative practice development. Every instance of practice is an act of faith with the ultimate but far-distant potential for internal healing and revolution. Each class is a contagious space in which transmission occurs not just through instruction, but also entrainment and mimicry. Each person is a colony of many voices, and intentions for the practice are easier to define than the governing agent that sets each intention. The processes of dwelling and crossing inherent in the development of yoga are echoed in the dwellings and crossings of each post-lineage practitioner, as they reach out from their existing sense of self to new spaces and new collaborations, to create new selves, and new ways of being at home (Tweed 2006: 75).

To do this, some practitioners take existing practices as given but modular elements, some reinterpret practices according to a perceived deeper purpose, and others seek divine, often 'feminine' inspiration. Some work towards an idealised, pristine self, others with the self as microbial temple, and others ritually construct oases of practice in which to explore intimacy and seek private truths. Some seek to confront the world, transform their own habits, and create resilience in disciplining the nervous system. Others dance with the moment-to-moment of experience, and sanctify their suffering. Post-lineage practice may be unusual but not unique in offering such opportunities for self-narration, self-reconciliation, self-empowerment and self-as-ecology. In the long, iterative process of turning personal revelation into shareable content, deeply intimate experiences of every possible mundane human suffering, from torn ligaments to chronic anxiety, are transformed by daily practice into narratives of hope and relief. As a result of such domestication of suffering into easily digestible stories of success, perhaps, following Carrette and King, the *shared* experience of post-lineage yoga is sometimes 'not quite troubling enough' (2013: 5). The hopeful stories and repeatable practices of post-lineage yoga teaching are a safe and comforting echo of what can arise within individual practice.

There are inherent risks to both individual and group practice, as a highly self-determined and yet intimately relational endeavour. Yet in transferring the practice to others, the risks and rewards of individual practice are, despite these safe stories, amplified. The deliberate connections made between physical and mental health, spiritual advancement, and world-changing action involve not just endless slippages between intention, outcome and side effect, but intensify the pressure on the practice to solve any possible personal problem. Post-lineage yoga does not wholly reconcile a troubled history of performativity, solipsism and universalism within modern postural yoga. It too slips perhaps too easily between training the body to external, geometric shapes, and finding shapes that conform to inner experience. And post-lineage yoga teachers largely still teach in person, performing the charisma of health in the form of physical exceptionality, or performing the narrative charisma of telling personal stories resonant with ancient magic.

The pragmatism of sharing the role of teacher, of being surrounded by peers, and of communal service, may temper the power of this charisma to unduly influence others. But the translation of the practice cycle to teaching environments, no matter how democratically organised or intuitively innovative, is as yet unevenly achieved. Post-lineage teaching, like its individual practice, is a highly semiogenetic process, in which meaning-making is entangled with inspiration and aspiration, charisma and catharsis. As a group movement practice, it is also complicated by powerful processes of mimesis that imbue bodily practice with hidden mechanisms of influence via association, empathy and metaphor. There can be an elision in the practice between the body or agency of the teacher and that of the student. It is not always clear in post-lineage yoga teaching whose experience is narrated, who decides the intention of practice and who decides the remedy for whom. In this book, I have noted some developments that seem to be useful in clarifying consent and agency during teaching, including invitational language, accessibility modifications, and protocols of consent. More work, and more research, in this area would be extremely useful.

POST-LINEAGE YOGA AS PART OF A GROWING REVOLUTION IN TRANSNATIONAL YOGA

Post-lineage yoga evolves out of modern postural yoga. Both exist on a spectrum where the former correlates to democratisation and student agency, and the latter to both the standardisation necessary for commercial success, and the hierarchies of knowledge associated with preserving existing practice through lineage. As this research project ends, significant changes in the institutions of contemporary yoga are taking place in numerous national contexts, affected by significant transnational forces. Here in Britain, the British Wheel of Yoga attempted to create national standards for yoga teaching to address what many teachers see as an epidemic of poorly trained teachers. This provoked significant criticism from the wider yoga teaching community, and contributed to the resignation of its own chair (BWY 2018). In America, independent studios are giving way to multinational brands, and the US-based Yoga Alliance has drawn criticism for a lack of oversight of training and teaching standards. Their own attempts to consult on new standards and a common scope of practice also provoked controversy, typified by Brown (2018), but both consultation and change still proceeded (Yoga Alliance UK 2018). The crisis in authority in contemporary transnational yoga continues to widen beyond individual lineages to affect governing bodies and professional organisations, and will undoubtedly include many more renegotiations in the authority to determine practice forms and meaning in yoga.

My findings clearly demonstrate that in Britain, at least, there is an intimate connection between post-lineage yoga practice, and the community network, subcultural norms and specific ecologies of its communal practice. Considering key trends in the history of yoga in Britain, including its engagement with local counterculture, the British context provides a unique and supportive environment for post-lineage yoga. Yoga here, like much of Europe, and in contrast with North America in particular, is disproportionately influenced by key charismatic figures who were against the totalising effects of yoga institutions, such as Krishnamurti (Goldberg 2016b: 74), Vanda Scaravelli (1991: 48), and Angela Farmer (Cummins 1997). Its core community, as represented by my case studies, continues that influence with their own shared suspicion of both commercialisation and standardisation. They also maintain overt and often shared involvements in political activism. Such radicalism, even when it is more of an ideal than a widespread practice, sets itself deliberately against a wider contemporary yoga culture that is considered by this subculture to be hopelessly apolitical, in its focus on individual rather than group empowerment, and its obsession with 'positive thinking' (Altglas 2014: 228).

Yoga's entry into the mainstream of British culture was also effected initially through adult education bodies that promoted standardisation, but also secularisation and democratisation (Newcombe 2013: 58). Despite the influence of local education initiatives, British yoga has no single organising body to mirror Yoga Alliance in the US. The commodification that seems inexorable and inescapable in analyses of American yoga (Strauss and Mandelbaum 2013: 177) seems thus far to be less prevalent in Britain. While in broad terms yoga in America is governed by entrepreneurial forces, in Britain, the constraining factors are arguably more bureaucratic in nature. But that bureaucracy has not led to significant standardisation or a single centralised authority. Further research may well discover that although the community of practice described by my research may be unusually coherent, post-lineage yoga, as a definitional attitude to teaching authority and student agency, is likely to apply to a great deal of teaching here in Britain.

Abuses by gurus within hierarchical lineages are, as I have shown, a common motivation for practitioners to start or join post-lineage communities of practice. Since this research began, revelations of abuse by respected yoga teachers are increasing in frequency and cultural relevance, in a conscious response to the #MeToo movement on social media (Carlson 2017; Rain 2018; Taylor 2018). Multiple allegations of abusive behaviours by perhaps the most well-known guru of modern yoga, Pattabhi Jois, such as in the twice-published article by Anneke Lucas (2016), and even visual records (yogagurusrevealed 2014; YogaDork 2009) have persisted for some years. Despite this, for many decades, and beyond Jois's death, Ashtanga Yoga has been one of the most enduring exemplars of guru worship in a modern postural yoga lineage.

But in the wake of Matthew Remski's very recent reframing of the stories of Jois's accusers (Remski 2018b), some Ashtanga Yoga teachers are attempting to evolve a more democratic and deliberately post-lineage authority structure. This can be evidenced by close reading of the rapidly evolving commentary of teachers such as Scott Johnson (2018), Anthony Grim Hall (2018) and Sarai Harvey Smith (2018), who are already calling for major changes to the Ashtanga Yoga teaching hierarchy. Some Ashtanga Yoga teachers are even using the term 'postlineage' as a hashtag to declare their independence from the Mysore teaching hierarchy. As this book goes to press, such profound changes appear to be part of a rising trend within transnational schools of yoga which will have unforeseeable effects in the years to come.

But beyond Britain, enumerating the prevalence of post-lineage subcultures must remain speculative at this point. In 2012 Katy Poole (2012) wrote an article on a well-regarded yoga-related site about the recent troubles in Anusara Yoga, with the prophetic conclusion that the era of 'the sage on the stage' in yoga was coming to an end. More recently, scholar Carol Horton's 'new paradigm' for contemporary yoga describes key aspects of a post-lineage approach (Horton 2018). Some transnational yoga communities seem more likely to embrace a post-lineage authority structure than others. It is unhelpful to associate the differences between lineage and post-lineage yoga with any perceived differences between what some might consider to be traditional and commodified forms. Standardisation and centralised authority are common, but not inevitable, in any yoga institution. There is much more correlation apparent between teachers of all forms of yoga who emphasise the agency and self-determination of the student, and those that embrace post-lineage authority structures. Teachers trained by Vanda Scaravelli, as I have shown, have often inherited from her a distrust of formal institutionalisation. The Desikachar-trained yoga community has similar tendencies, and has been involved in numerous struggles with the institutionalisation of authority, as shown in statements by Paul Harvey (2013) and Leslie Kaminoff (2018). Some commodified yoga brands such as Bikram Choudhury's Bikram Yoga on the other hand are extremely authoritarian in the prescription of both practice and teaching protocols (Friedman 2015; Healy 2015; Jain 2012: 7).

It can be argued that lineage, as its role is understood in modern postural yoga, developed in close relationship to commodification and modernism (Sarbacker 2014: 108) just as it developed in close relationship with Indian independence and postcolonialism, from pre-modern precedents in ascetic lineages (Singleton 2013: 45). The major transnational lineages are as much brands or family businesses as religious lineages (Krishna 2016). What is often considered to be traditional, lineage-based yoga, is also shaped by the forces of modernity. There is no clear line to neatly separate them from the secularised, commodified yoga of brands, nor from the lineages of pre-modern history (Sarbacker 2014: 109–10). Beyond the practice sanctioned by major lineages, ashrams and historical texts, as historians of yoga seek to understand the vernacular precedents and historical authority structures of postural practice (Broo 2015), there may be a very different picture to emerge of the forms of yoga that have been shared historically in local communities across South Asia, outside of institutions. While specific historical communities probably drew from a narrower repertoire than is available to most contemporary practitioners, there may be many such small-scale scenes or subcultures (Moberg and Ramstedt 2016: 160), themselves made up of overlapping communities of practice.

Contemporary yoga is a global practice that includes great cultural diversity, but it also supports a number of extremely profitable international industries (Lavrence and Lozanski 2014: 77; Goldberg 2015; Hauser 2013a: 6). The marketing of innumerable health-related products use yoga-related imagery (Puustinen and Rautaniemi 2015: 48). Yoga clothing mega-brand Lululemon reports sales of over $900 million a quarter (Shaw 2018). Yet none of these industries contribute to the financial stability of yoga teachers in any country, beyond a few highly paid, international celebrity teachers. Yoga teaching for the majority is described as increasingly competitive and poorly paid (Goldberg 2015). And seeking to govern this grassroots, chaotically diverse, often female-led enterprise of teaching yoga, are a number of mostly male, mostly white business graduates (Jaqueline Hargreaves, personal communication, 2018). In this regard, much of the rest of the world differs from America only in degree.

In various national and international contexts, bureaucrats, lineages, brands, new media platforms, scholars, practitioners, and governments, are currently struggling to define and thus control yoga. The separation of contemporary yoga actors into yoga-consuming industries, regulating bureaucracies, and practice-producing communities is a useful generalisation to employ here. If we are to determine that which governs contemporary yoga on a transnational scale, it is vital to delineate the relevant structures of power and profit. The right to profit from yoga, can include the right to define it. And as older systems of patriarchal, institutionalised authority within yoga are breaking down, the emerging calls to professionalise or regulate yoga teaching from any quarter are in fact unlikely to safeguard the future of yoga teachers, but might instead reduce vital diversity, and increase the economic insecurity of the practice community (Hargreaves 2018: 4).

But post-lineage yoga, in any form, has thus far provided no systematic justice for survivors of abuse by charismatic teachers, and few safe spaces for community building online (Howard 2013: 83). It is possible that as a form of transmission, it does not scale well beyond small, in-person networks. Nor does the valuable peer support offered by such networks negate the vulnerable position of many teachers within the now-endemic and precarious 'gig economy'. Nonetheless, the yoga practice of the sort shared here provides for many, one of a number of similar practices, also used as imperfect answers to rising levels of social isolation, anxiety and exhaustion (hooks 2016; Rosa 2004: 697). This may be a practice promoting localised resilience and service (Oh and Sarkisian 2012: 315), if not one that empowers social reform.

FURTHER RISKS, OPPORTUNITIES AND IMPLICATIONS FOR THE FUTURE

Much of the future transmission of post-lineage yoga as a practice may depend on whether it will retain the flexibility of currently evolving peer-networked authority, and also honour the depth of powerful meaning-making inherent in current iterations of the practice, even as it responds to new socio-political pressures and growing demands for 'safe' practice spaces. Any large national or even transnational organisation of yoga teachers that wishes to support the ongoing evolution of post-lineage yoga would do well to consider itself as a diverse federation of linked subcultures, local scenes and communities, grounded in the creativity of real-world crossings and dwellings. If so, post-lineage networks will retain their role in ensuring the resilience and localisation of contemporary yoga practice.

When the majority of those engaged in that localisation are white Anglophones, such as here in Britain, the tangled history of colonial oppression in South Asia continues to hold some influence over that process. This book does not contribute significantly to that debate, and I prefer to defer to Indian and diasporic voices in that regard. But in India, yoga teaching has historically been a vehicle for political struggles in caste and class relationships, against colonialism, and for the development of a newly independent national identity. The current nationalist government continues that long history by devoting increasing resources to the global promotion of a specifically Indian and Hindu yoga as a form of political soft power (Black 2016: 29; Hauser 2013a: 6). As an unfortunate side effect, social media debates about authenticity in yoga practice have, in recent years, seen a troubling rise in anti-intellectualism and the essentialisation of Indian religious identities, as detailed by Jain (2014b) and Patankar (2014), and exemplified by Reynolds (2015).

New media technologies enable many of the interpersonal conversations at the heart of yoga peer networking, but also more fraught, even aggressive interactions between yoga subcultures with very different values and priorities (Horton 2015, 2016). The targeted trolling of prominent writers, public figures and scholars of yoga such as myself, for political or personal gain, is becoming an ingrained problem across social media platforms. In the public conversations among teachers of all forms of contemporary yoga, tensions between orthopraxy, commodification, and international politics, are intensifying.

Like any similar academic endeavour, this research seeks only to describe, not bestow approval upon the phenomenon of post-lineage yoga. Yet for many who have become uncomfortable with self-definitions grounded in lineage, brand, or other institutional identity, the label of post-lineage yoga is an opportunity to discover themselves as part of a trend beyond their immediate community of practice. For those most threatened by the recognition of any yoga subculture with grassroots approaches to recognising authority and authenticity however, the term is immediately threatening, and provokes aggressive responses and malicious misinterpretation. It is in that context that this book will be published.

FINAL THOUGHTS

Beyond the methodology, the understudied subculture, and the wider processes of negotiated authority set out herein, this book is a response to previous academic assumptions concerning religious practice, the shared construction of meaning, performative agency, and religious henotheism and consumerism. It attempts to move debates about yoga as religious practice from embodied mindfulness to animated bodies, from institutions to vernacular communities, from the universal to the diverse. Within this book, multiple possible definitions of yoga: as repeated method; as a focus of discipline; as aim, intention or state, and as shared subculture and repertoire, are all addressed. My aim has been, above all, to highlight the difference between the individuality and secularity of discourses surrounding contemporary yoga, and the often communal, ritual nature of its actual lived experience (Nye 2000: 458). Ritualised movement practices such as post-lineage yoga are part of the meaning-making that human beings choose to create, to enact and to experience (Spickard 2005: 354). This is where the *creation* of meaning, and the *re-enactment* of meaning, meet. At the heart of post-lineage yoga practice are visceral memories, movement as self-creation, and flesh shaped through action.

As my focus throughout has been to amplify unheard stories, I am however aware of how many of the stories of contemporary yoga and other similar practices are left to be told. Modern yoga research, particularly the anthropological study of yoga, would greatly benefit from significant investigation into such experiences as: the lived history of yoga practitioners of colour; the motivations of those who have left the practice behind; more diverse Indian and diasporic voices on yoga (Spivak 2008: 79); and the experiences of those vulnerable populations using yoga to innovative ends, particularly trauma survivors, prison populations and disabled students.

Only the extremely privileged have the possibility of considering their physical existence to be normal, stable, or safe. The rest survive through reconciliation with the body we are, with all its wounds and healings, imposed habits and transformations. It is possible to consider all the diverse practices of contemporary and historical yoga as responses to different forms of suffering, in keeping with many other religious practices. To the extent that they are technologies of liberation, they are never apolitical or disembodied. Bodies in yoga move, breathe, align and transform. Bodies in yoga are colonised and decolonised, commercialised, sanitised and reclaimed, in contested space. Under the skin of *āsana* and *prāṇāyāma*, *pratyahara* and *kīrtan*, politics, pain, joy and belief are mattered in flesh.

The most significant transmission innovation of yoga in the modern era may well be practising as a group, and yet both scholars, and teacher-practitioners, are only just beginning to understand what it means for bodies to practise this most intimate of arts together. Without patronage or orthodox approval, without academic or public visibility, scattered and networked across time and space, post-lineage practitioners are already finding, teaching, and supporting each other.

Finally, and most clearly, at the heart of post-lineage yoga are practitioners mimicking a long heritage of predecessors in the imperfect attempt to create an emplaced, embodied counter-practice to the pressures of their time. With the right allies, the right framing, and the right practice, they hope that the individual and group bodies that emerge might be less easy to predict, to control, and to market. Theirs is a spiralling technology of individual practice and group entrainment. It maps the many layers of the self-world in accordance with an ever-evolving repertoire of movement and stillness. Above all, post-lineage yoga continues to take place off the mat and in the world, even as the practitioner dreams of transcendence, of silence, and of reconciliation.

GLOSSARY

Yoga

A practice of self-conscious, ritualised movement and stillness, focused on somatic or sensory experience, set within subcultures that are linked to diverse beliefs and engaged in complex relationships with the religions and cultures of the Indian sub-continent.

Post-lineage yoga

Subcultures of yoga practice in which teachers and practitioners that have rejected or been ostracised from their lineage of study come together in peer-to-peer networks to evolve and share yoga practice with others who maintain allegiance to a lineage, but look beyond it as the sole authority to determine practice.

INDIC TERMS

āsana	Originally 'seat', refers to the postures and movements of physical practice
bhakti	Practices of devotion, commonly including *sevā* and *kīrtan*
haṭhayoga	A collection of practices that traditionally includes *āsana*, *prāṇāyāma* and meditation, for much of its history associated with certain anti-social behaviours, reclaimed as the foundation of modern postural yoga
kīrtan	Devotional singing, often in call and response form
kriyā	Cleansing practices that can overlap in form with *āsana* or *prāṇāyāma*
mantra	Repetitive chanting with devotional or magical intent
mudrā	Ritualised hand gesture for devotional or magical intent
mūrti	Representation of a divine being that is also a living embodiment of the same
prāṇāyāma	Practices of breath observation and/or control
pūjā	Devotional ritual consisting of chants and offerings made to figures on an altar

sevā	Devotional service, originally to the guru, now with a diversity of communal or humanitarian targets
yoganidrā	A form of guided deep relaxation originally developed from an esoteric Tantric technique known as *nyāsa*

TECHNICAL TERMS

entrainment	Often unconscious synchronisation of organic movement such as gesture and heart rate to an external rhythm
interoception	Awareness of one's internal physiological condition
kinetic	Pertaining to movement
mimesis	Physical imitation, mimicry
semiogenesis or semiogenetic	Meaning-making or productive of meaning
sensorimotor	Involving both sensory and motor activity, such as sensorimotor amnesia, the partial and uneven loss of bodily sensation and movement through trauma or disuse
somatic	Pertaining to the senses

KEY PEOPLE AND EVENTS

Christopher	Case study 1, teacher of Engaged Yoga
Ian	Co-founder of the One Spirit Ashram Kitchen
Nicole	Case study 6, teacher of Soma Yoga
Robbie	Co-organiser of Colourfest
Rowan	Co-organiser of Colourfest
Sivani Mata	Case study 4, *bhakti* musician and teacher of Womb Yoga and Shakti Dance
Tanya	Case study 5, co-organiser of Sundara with her husband John
Trishula	Organiser of the Beltane Bhakti Gathering
Uma	Case study 3, organiser of Santosa
Veronika	Case study 1, teacher of Reflex Yoga

Colourfest	Colourfest festival
Santosa	Santosa Living Yoga and Bhakti Camp
Sundara	Sundara Community Gathering

SUBCULTURAL INFLUENCES

Ashtanga (Vinyasa) Yoga	A specific *āsana* and *vinyāsa* based practice fixed during the Mysore modern yoga revival by Pattabhi Jois
(Sri Haidakhandi) Babaji	One of numerous Hindu saints known as Babaji
British Wheel of Yoga	The most secular and normative of governing institutions in the UK, it has links to Iyengar Yoga, various LEAs and Skills Active
Divine feminine	A school of feminist religious thought, with associated yoga forms that focus on female representation and practices appropriate for female bodies, exemplified by Angela Farmer and Vanda Scaravelli
Hatha Yoga	Designation often used when a yoga practice is outside the most common and visible lineages, sometimes used to designate a gentler practice form
Independent Yoga Network	The most independent and smallest of the three main yoga governing institutions in the UK
Integral Yoga	Yoga practice inspired by and developed from the teachings of Swami Satchidananda, promoting the holistic integration of spiritual activities
Iyengar Yoga	Corrective, therapeutic and *āsana*-based practice for health that closely follows the teachings of BKS Iyengar, part of the Mysore yoga revival
Kundalini Yoga	Yoga practice inspired by and developed from the teachings of Yogi Bhajan, focused on esoteric development and raising *kuṇḍalinī*
Reflex Yoga	Therapeutic yoga techniques developed by Veronika de la Pena and Nicole Zimbler from lay understandings of infant neurology
Satyananda Yoga	Tantra-derived yoga practices inspired by the teachings of Swami Satyananda

Scaravelli Inspired Yoga	There is a loose school of 'divine feminine' yoga practices inspired by the lifework of Vanda Scaravelli, who asked her students not to name a school after her. 'Scaravelli Inspired' is a self-chosen label that expresses a teacher's compromise between honouring that request and the need to signal the kind of approach they use in teaching
Shakti Dance	Kundalini Yoga inspired combination of yoga and dance
Sivananda Yoga	Patañjali-inspired yoga practice developed from the teachings of Swami Sivananda
Total Yoga Nidra Network	Learning community of post-lineage *yoganidrā* teachers co-founded by Uma Dinsmore-Tuli and her husband, Nirlipta Tuli
Vipassana	Popular Buddhist form of meditation including Anapana (breath awareness), systematic bodily observation and the cultivation of equanimity
Womb Yoga	Contemporary yoga school emphasising seasonal rhythms and the divine feminine developed by Uma Dinsmore-Tuli
Yoga Alliance	Voluntary but dominant body for accrediting yoga teaching in the US, with an increasingly international reach
Yoga Alliance Professionals, formerly Yoga Alliance UK	The most commercial of governing institutions in the UK, with no formal connection to Yoga Alliance

REFERENCES

Aarons, Nicole. 2017. 'Soma Yoga and Medicine School (Facebook Status Update)', retrieved 9 May 2017 from www.facebook.com/soma.hummingbird/posts/1843400119253819.

Adams, Jimi. 2013. 'Network Analysis', in Michael Stausberg and Steven Engler (eds), *The Routledge Handbook of Research Methods in the Study of Religion* (Routledge: London).

Alter, Joseph S. 2005. 'Modern Medical Yoga: Struggling with a History of Magic, Alchemy and Sex', *Asian Medicine*, 1: 119–46.

——. 2006. 'Yoga at the Fin de Siècle: Muscular Christianity with a "Hindu" Twist', *The International Journal of the History of Sport*, 23: 759–76.

——. 2012. 'Sacrifice, the Body, and Yoga: Theoretical Entailments of Embodiment in Hathayoga', *South Asia-Journal of South Asian Studies*, 35: 408–33.

Altglas, Véronique. 2014. *From yoga to Kabbalah: Religious Exoticism and the Logics of Bricolage* (Oxford University Press: New York).

Apperley, Alan. 2014. 'Revisiting Dearing: Higher Education and the Construction of the 'Belabored' Self', *Culture Unbound: Journal of Current Cultural Research*, 6: 731–54.

Apperley, Alan, Stephen Jacobs, and Mark Jones. 2014. 'Introduction: Therapeutic Culture', *Culture Unbound: Journal of Current Cultural Research*, 6: 725–29.

Armstrong, Clairette. 1953. 'Some Notes on Imagery in Psychophysical Therapy', *Journal of General Psychology*, 49: 231.

Athreya, Preethi. 2001. 'Making Dance: A Choreological Approach', retrieved 14 August 2018 from www.narthaki.com/info/articles/article66.html.

Aune, Kristin. 2011. 'Much Less Religious, a Little More Spiritual: The Religious and Spiritual Views of Third-Wave Feminists in the UK', *Feminist Review*: 32–55.

Baistow, Karen. 1994. 'Liberation and Regulation? Some Paradoxes of Empowerment', *Critical Social Policy*, 14: 34–46.

Baker, Lindsay. 2015. 'Why Music Festivals Won't Die', retrieved 26 September 2017 from www.bbc.com/culture/story/20150622-why-music-festivals-wont-die.

Barsalou, Lawrence, Aron Barbey, W. Kyle Simmons, and Ava Santos. 2005. 'Embodiment in Religious Knowledge', *Journal of Cognition and Culture*, 5: 14–57.

Bauwens, Michel. 2014. 'If we Can Have P2P Economics, Why Not P2P Spirituality?', retrieved 7 December 2018 from www.opendemocracy.net/transformation/michel-bauwens/if-we-can-have-p2p-economics-why-not-p2p-spirituality.

Beckerlegge, Gwilym. 2011. 'Seva (Service to Humanity): A Boundary Issue in The Study of Recent and Contemporary Hindu Movements', *Man in India*, 91: 39–56.

——. 2015. 'Seva: The Focus of a Fragmented but Gradually Coalescing Field of Study', *Religions of South Asia*, 9: 208–39.

Behnke, Elizabeth A. 1997. 'Ghost Gestures: Phenomenological Investigations of Bodily Micromovements and their Intercorporeal Implications', *Human Studies*, 20: 181–201.

Bender, Courtney. 2012. 'Practicing Religions', in Robert A. Orsi (ed.), *The Cambridge Companion to Religious Studies* (Cambridge University Press: Cambridge).

Bennett, Jane. 2002. *Thoreau's Nature: Ethics, Politics, and the Wild* (Rowman & Littlefield: Lanham).

Bhajan, Yogi. 2008a. 'For Healing Addictions', retrieved 15 May 2017 from www.3ho.org/files/documents/forhealingaddictions.pdf.

——. 2008b. 'Kundalini Yoga', retrieved 15 May 2017 from www.3ho.org.

——. 2017. 'Sodarshan Chakra Kriya', retrieved 9 May 2017 from www.3ho.org/kundalini-yoga/teaching/sodarshan-chakra-kriya.

Birch, Jason. 2011. 'The Meaning of Hatha in Early Hathayoga', *Journal of the American Oriental Society*, 4: 527–54.

——. 2016. 'The Haṭha Yoga Project (a Talk Presented at the British Museum, April 2016)', retrieved 11 March 2017 from www.academia.edu/24233544/The_Ha%E1%B9%ADha_Yoga_Project_a_Talk_Presented_at_the_British_Museum_April_2016_?auto=download.

Birch, Jason, and Jaqueline Hargreaves. 2015a. 'Extending the Breath to Defeat Death', retrieved 17 December 2015 from http://theluminescent.blogspot.in/2015/12/December extending-breath-to-defeat-death.html.

——. 2015b. 'Yoganidra: An Understanding of the History and Context', retrieved 6 January 2015 from http://theluminescent.blogspot.fr/2015/01/yoganidra.html.

——. 2016. 'The Yamas and Niyamas: Medieval and Modern Views', *Yoga Scotland*, retrieved 4 June 2020 from www.academia.edu/25130842/The_Yamas_and_Niyamas_Part_2_-_Medieval_and_Modern_Views

Birney, Bernadette. 2016. 'Joint Hypermobility Syndrome: Yoga's Enigmatic Epidemic?', retrieved 4 February 2016 from https://yogainternational.com/article/view/joint-hypermobility-syndrome-yogas-enigmatic-epidemic.

Black, Shameem. 2016. 'Flexible Indian Labor: Yoga, Information Technology Migration, and U.S. Technoculture', *Race and Yoga*, 1: 22–39.

Blackaby, Peter. 2016. 'Yoga and the Mereological Fallacy', retrieved 28 June 16 from www.intelligentyoga.co.uk/yoga-and-the-mereological-fallacy.

——. 2018. 'Intelligent Yoga', paper presented at The Future of Yoga, 2018 IYN Conference, Wolverhampton, UK.

Blair, Norman. 2017. *Brightening Our Inner Skies: Yin and Yoga* (MicMac Margins: London).

Blevins, John. 2008. 'Different Subjects: Postmodern Selves in Psychology and Religion', *Pastoral Psychology*, 57: 25–44.

Blomberg, Harald. 2015. *The Rhythmic Movement Method: A Revolutionary Approach to Improved Health and Well-Being* (Lulu Publishing Services: Morrisville).

Bowman, Marion. 2009. 'Learning from Experience: The Value of Analysing Avalon', *Religion*, 39: 161–68.

Broad, William J. 2012. *The Science of Yoga: The Risks and the Rewards* (Simon & Schuster: Bath).

Brom, Danny, Yaffa Stokar, Cathy Lawi, Vered Nuriel-Porat, Yuval Ziv, Karen Lerner, and Gina Ross. 2017. 'Somatic Experiencing for Posttraumatic Stress Disorder: A Randomized Controlled Outcome Study', *Journal of Traumatic Stress*, 30: 304–12.

Broo, Måns. 2015. 'Hinduism and the Question of Founders', in Patrick Gray (ed.), *Varieties of Religious Invention: Founders and Their Functions in History* (Oxford University Press: Oxford).

Brosi, George. 2012. 'The Beloved Community: A Conversation with bell hooks', *Appalachian Heritage*, 40.

Brown, Christina. 2009. *The Yoga Bible: The Definitive Guide to Yoga Postures* (Godsfield: London).

Brown, Jason. 2015. 'Am I Misappropriating Yoga?', retrieved 3 November 2015 from www.jbrownyoga.com/blog/2015/11/am-i-misappropriating-yoga?mc_cid=80bf64055a&mc_eid=68a7a1c421.

——. 2017a. 'Getting Off the Crack', retrieved 11 March 2017 from www.jbrown yoga.com/blog/2017/3/getting-off-the-crack.

——. 2017b. 'Theo Wildcroft – "Wild Yoga" – Doctoral Researcher, Yoga Teacher, lover of vulnerable people and wild things', retrieved 15 February 2017 from www.jbrownyoga.com/yoga-talks-podcast/2017/2/theo-wildcroft.

——. 2018. 'Andrew Tanner – "Standards Review" – Yoga Alliance Chief Advancement Officer, Standards Review Project Survey', retrieved 4 June 2020 from www.jbrownyoga.com/yoga-talks-podcast/2018/2/andrew-tanner

Bubandt, Nils, and Rane Willerslev. 2015. 'The Dark Side of Empathy: Mimesis, Deception, and the Magic of Alterity', *Comparative Studies in Society and History*, 57: 5–34.

Burger, Maya. 2006. 'What Price Salvation? The Exchange of Salvation Goods between India and the West', *Social Compass*, 53: 81–95.

Burley, Mikel. 2014. '"A Petrification of One's Own Humanity"?Nonattachment and Ethics in Yoga Traditions', *Journal of Religion*, 94: 204–28.

BWY. 2018. 'Statement from the NEC', retrieved 14 May 2018 from www.bwy.org.uk/news–90.

Caldarelli, Guido, and Michele Catanzaro. 2012. *Networks: A Very Short Introduction* (Oxford University Press: Oxford).

Carlson, Karin. 2017. 'Yoga and #metoo: We Can Do Better', retrieved 29 January 2018 from http://yogadork.com/2017/12/17/yoga-and-metoo-we-can-do-better.

Carp, Richard M. 2001. 'Integrative Praxes: Learning from Multiple Knowledge Formations', *Issues in Integrative Studies*, 19: 71–121.

Carrette, Jeremy R., and Richard King. 2013. *Selling Spirituality: The Silent Takeover of Religion* (Routledge: London).

Carrier, James. 1991. 'Gifts, Commodities, and Social-Relations – a Maussian View of Exchange', *Sociological Forum*, 6: 119–36.

Castells, Manuel. 2011. 'A Network Theory of Power', *International Journal of Communications*, 5: 773–87.

Chryssides, George D. 2012. 'The New Age', in Mikael Rothstein and Olav Hammer (eds), *The Cambridge Companion to New Religious Movements* (Cambridge University Press: Cambridge).

Cixous, Hélène. 1976. 'Laugh of the Medusa', *Signs*, 1: 875–93.

Cixous, Hélène, and Susan Sellers. 1994. *The Hélène Cixous reader* (Routledge: London).

Clark, David. 1996. 'The Community Educator', in, *Schools As Learning Communities: Transforming Education* (Cassell: London).

Cole, Johnathan, and Barbara Montero. 2007. 'Affective Proprioception', *Janus Head*, 9: 299–317.

Coleman, Mathew, and Kevin Grove. 2009. 'Biopolitics, Biopower, and the Return of Sovereignty', *Environment and Planning D: Society and Space*, 27: 489–507.

Compson, Jane. 2014. 'Meditation, Trauma and Suffering in Silence: Raising Questions about How Meditation is Taught and Practiced in Western Contexts in the Light of a Contemporary Trauma Resiliency Model', *Contemporary Buddhism*, 15: 274–97.

Consultancy.uk. 2017. 'Top 10 Largest Music Festivals in the UK', retrieved 16 July 2019 from www.consultancy.uk/news/13576/top-10-largest-music-festivals-in-the-uk.

Cope, Stephen. 1999. *Yoga and the Quest for the True Self* (Bantam Books: New York).

Crockford, Susannah. 2017. 'After the American Dream: The Political Economy of spirituality in Northern Arizona, USA', The London School of Economics and Political Science.

Cuffari, Elena, Ezequiel Paolo, and Hanne Jaegher. 2015. 'From Participatory Sense-making to Language: There and Back Again', *Phenomenology and the Cognitive Sciences*, 14: 1089–125.

Cummins, Claudia. 1997. 'Angela Farmer – The Feminine Unfolding', retrieved 29 March 2016 from www.youtube.com/watch?v=soA-PHxcgbI.

Da'oud, Emilie C. 1995. 'Life on Land', in Don Johnson (ed.), *Bone, Breath & Gesture : Practices of Embodiment* (North Atlantic Books: Berkeley).

———. 1997. 'Continuum', in Don Johnson (ed.), *Groundworks : Narratives of Embodiment* (North Atlantic Books: Berkeley).

Dark Mountain Project. 2010. *Dark Mountain* (Dark Mountain Project: Croydon).

Davies, Andy. 2013. 'Re-imagining Communities of Practice: Does this Underpin Modern Yoga Teacher Training?', *International Journal of Pedagogies & Learning*, 8: 39–44.

De Michelis, Elizabeth. 2007. 'A Preliminary Survey of Modern Yoga Studies', *Asian Medicine*, 3: 1–19.

de Waal, Frans B. M. 2008. 'Putting the Altruism Back into Altruism: The Evolution of Empathy', in, *Annual Review of Psychology* (Annual Reviews: Palo Alto).

——. 2012. 'A Bottom-up View of Empathy', in Frans B. M. de Waal and Pier Francesco Ferrari (eds), *The Primate Mind: Built to Connect with Other Minds*. (Harvard University Press: Harvard).

Ded, Lalla, and Ranjit Hoskote. 2013. *I, Lalla: The Poems of Lal Ded* (Penguin: New York).

Depraz, Natalie. 2008. 'The Rainbow of Emotions: At the Crossroads of Neurobiology and Phenomenology', *Continental Philosophy Review*, 41: 237–59.

Deslippe, Philip. 2012. 'From Maharaj to Mahan Tantric: The construction of Yogi Bhajan's Kundalini Yoga', *Sikh Formations*, 8: 369–87.

Devi, Nischala J. 2010. *The Secret Power of Yoga: A Woman's Guide to the Heart and Spirit of the Yoga Sutras* (Crown Publishing: New York).

Devine, Megan. 2015. 'Everything is not Okay' from www.refugeingrief.com/support/audiobook.

Dharma, Vishwa Nirmala. 2017. 'Sahaja Yoga', retrieved 9 May 2017 from www.sahajayoga.org.

Dinsmore-Tuli, Uma. 2013a. 'Santosa: The Inside Story', retrieved 20 September 2016 from www.santosayogacamp.co.uk/content/santosa-inside-story.

——. 2013b. *Yoni Shakti: A Woman's Guide to Power and Freedom Through Yoga and Tantra* (Yogawords: London).

Dinsmore-Tuli, Uma, and Jack Harrison. 2015. *The Celtic School of Yoga: An Aisling for the 21st Century* (The Celtic School of Yoga: Kinvara).

Dinsmore-Tuli, Uma, and Nirlipta Tuli. 2018a. 'Free Yoga Nidras', retrieved 28 May 2018 from www.yoganidranetwork.org/downloads.

——. 2018b. 'Online Learning', retrieved 28 May 2018 from www.yoganidranetwork.org/online-learning.

——. 2018c. 'Total Yoga Nidra and Swami Satyananda: where we stand now', retrieved 17 January 2018 from www.yoganidranetwork.org/article/total-yoga-nidra-and-swami-satyananda-where-we-stand-now.

Doniger, Wendy. 2013. *On Hinduism* (Oxford University Press: Oxford).

Dreyfus, Hubert. 1996. 'The Current Relevance of Merleau-Ponty's Phenomenology of Embodiment', *The Electronic Journal of Analytic Philosophy*, 4.

Emerson, David, and Elizabeth Hopper. 2012. *Overcoming Trauma through Yoga: Reclaiming Your Body* (North Atlantic Books: Berkeley, CA).

Encyclopædia Britannica. 2016. 'Esoteric', retrived 4 June 2020 from www.britannica.com/topic/esotericism

Falk, Geoffrey D. 2009. *Stripping the Gurus: Sex, Violence, Abuse and Enlightenment* (Million Monkeys Press: New York).

Featherstone, Mike. 2010. 'Body, Image and Affect in Consumer Culture', *Body and Society*, 16: 193–221.

Fleischman, Paul R. 2016. *You Can Never Speak Up Too Often for the Love of All Things* (Pariyatti Publishing: Onalaska, WA).

Foldy, Erica G. 2004. 'Learning from Diversity: A Theoretical Exploration', *Public Administration Review*, 64: 529–29.

Fraleigh, Sondra H. 2000. 'Conciousness Matters', *Dance Research Journal*, 32: 54.

Francis, Sivani Mata. 2017. 'Jasmine Garden', retrieved 4 June 2020 from https://sivanimata.bandcamp.com/album/jasmine-garden

Freire, Paulo. 1996. *Pedagogy of the Oppressed* (Penguin: London).

Freschi, Elisa, and Philipp A. Maas. 2016. 'Introduction: Conceptual Reflections on Adaptive Reuse' in Elisa Freschi and Philipp A. Maas (eds), *Adaptive Reuse: Aspects of Creativity in South Asian Cultural History* (Harrassowitz Verlag: Wiesbaden).

Friedman, Jennifer. 2015. 'What the Bikram Copyright Rejection Means for Yoga', retrieved 7 July 2017 from www.yogajournal.com/lifestyle/rejection-bikram-copyright-upheld-means-future-yoga?_escaped_fragment_=.

Gaard, Greta. 2001. 'Tools for a Cross-Cultural Feminist Ethics: Exploring Ethical Contexts and Contents in the Makah', *Hypatia*, 16: 1.

——. 2010. 'New Directions for Ecofeminism: Toward a More Feminist Ecocriticism', *Isle-Interdisciplinary Studies in Literature and Environment*, 17: 643–65.

Geeves, Andrew, Doris J. F. McIlwain, John Sutton, and Wayne Christensen. 2014. 'To Think or Not To Think: The Apparent Paradox of Expert Skill in Music Performance', *Educational Philosophy and Theory*, 46: 674–91.

Giardina, Michael D., and Joshua I. Newman. 2011. 'Physical Cultural Studies and Embodied Research Acts', *Cultural Studies ↔ Critical Methodologies*, 11: 523–34.

Gilman, Sander L. 2014. '"Stand up Straight": Notes toward a History of Posture', *The Journal of Medical Humanities*, 35: 57.

Ginot, Isabelle. 2010. 'From Shusterman's Somaesthetics to a Radical Epistemology of Somatics', *Dance Research Journal*, 42: 12–29.

Gladwell, Christopher, and Louise Wender. 2014. *Engaged Yoga* (Siddha Publishing: [Bristol?]).

Glassie, Henry. 1995. 'Tradition', *Journal of American Folklore*, 108: 395–412.

Glendening, Daniel. 2012. 'ECCC12 Edward James Olmos Inspires With Humility', retrieved 29 January 2018 from www.cbr.com/eccc12-edward-james-olmos-inspires-with-humility.

Godrej, Farah. 2012. 'Ascetics, Warriors, and a Gandhian Ecological Citizenship', *Political Theory*, 40: 437–65.

Goldberg, Eliott. 2016a. *The Path of Modern Yoga: The History of an Embodied Spiritual Practice* (Inner Traditions: Rochester).

Goldberg, Michelle. 2015. 'The Brutal Economics of Being a Yoga Teacher', retrieved 7 December 2017 from http://nymag.com/thecut/2015/10/brutal-economics-of-being-a-yoga-teacher.html.

——. 2016b. *The Goddess Pose: The Audacious Life of Indra Devi, the Woman Who Helped Bring Yoga to the West* (Corsair: London).

Goodenough, Anne E., Natasha Little, William S. Carpenter, and Adam G. Hart. 2017. 'Birds of a Feather Flock Together: Insights into Starling Murmuration Behaviour Revealed Using Citizen Science', *Plos One*, 12: 18.

Graziano, Michael S. A. 2016. 'Ethological Action Maps: A Paradigm Shift for the Motor Cortex', *Trends in Cognitive Sciences*, 20: 121–32.

Grimes, Ronald L. 1995. *Beginnings in Ritual Studies* (University of South Carolina Press: Columbia).

Guest, Ann Hutchinson. 2007. *An introduction to motif notation* (Language of Dance Centre: London).

Gura, Phillip F. 2006. 'A Wild, Rank Place', in Joel Myerson (ed.), *The Cambridge Companion to Henry David Thoreau* (Cambridge University Press: Cambridge).

Hall, Anthony Grim. 2018. 'No Longer Identifying as an Ashtangi ... or a 'yogi' for that Matter', retrieved 4 June 2018 from https://grimmly2007.blogspot.com/2018/06/no-longer-identifying-as-ashtangi-or.html.

Harding, Walter. 2006. 'Thoreau's Reputation', in Joel Myerson (ed.), *The Cambridge Companion to Henry David Thoreau* (Cambridge University Press: Cambridge).

Hargreaves, Jaqueline. 2017. 'Postural Punishment in Indian Schools', retrieved 15 January 201 from http://theluminescent.blogspot.co.uk/2017/01/postural-punishment-in-indian-schools.html.

———. 2018. 'Yoga Alliance is Dead, Long Live Yoga (Alliance?)', retrieved 13 March 2018 from https://theluminescent.blogspot.co.uk/2018/02/yoga-alliance-is-dead-long-live-yoga.html.

Hart, William. 2011. *The Art of Living: Vipassana Meditation as Taught by S. N. Goenka* (Pariyatti Publishing: Onalaska, WA).

Harvey, Graham. 2006. *Animism : Respecting the Living World* (Columbia University Press: New York).

———. 2012. 'Rituals in New Religions', in Mikael Rothstein and Olav Hammer (eds), *The Cambridge Companion to New Religious Movements* (Cambridge University Press: Cambridge).

———. 2014. *Food, Sex and Strangers: Understanding Religion as Everyday Life* (Routledge: London).

Harvey, Paul. 2013. 'Viniyoga', retrieved 13 March 2018 from www.yogastudies.org/sanskrit/viniyoga.

Hasselle-Newcombe, Suzanne. 2005. 'Spirituality and 'Mystical Religion' in Contemporary Society: A Case Study of British Practitioners of the Iyengar Method of Yoga', *Journal of Contemporary Religion*, 20: 305–21.

Haugen, Sigrid Steen. 2016. 'Moving and Feeling – An Exploration of the Play between Motion, Emotion and Motivation in Yoga Practitioners in Norway', Norwegian University of Science and Technology.

Hauser, Beatrix. 2013a. 'Introduction: Transcultural Yoga(s). Analyzing a Traveling Subject', in Beatrix Hauser (ed.), *Yoga Traveling: Bodily Practice in Transcultural Perspective* (Springer International Publishing: New York).

———. 2013b. 'Touching the Limits, Assessing Pain: On Language Performativity, Health, and Well-Being in Yoga Classes ' in Beatrix Hauser (ed.), *Yoga Traveling: Bodily Practice in Transcultural Perspective* (Springer International Publishing: New York).

Healy, Jack. 2015. 'Schism Emerges in Bikram Yoga Empire Amid Rape Claims' from www.nytimes.com/2015/02/24/us/cracks-show-in-bikram-yoga-empire-amid-claims-of-rape-and-assault.html.

Hebdige, Dick. 1979. *Subculture: The Meaning of Style* (Routledge: New York).

Heelas, Paul. 1993. 'The New Age in Cultural Context: The Premodern, the Modern and the Postmodern', *Religion*, 23: 103–16.

Hervieu-Léger, Danièle. 2000. *Religion as a Chain of Memory* (Rutgers University Press: New Brunswick).

Holloway, Julian. 2003. 'Make-Believe: Spiritual Practice, Embodiment, and Sacred Space', *Environment and Planning A*, 35: 1961–74.

hooks, bell. 1989. 'Choosing the Margin as Space of Radical Openness', *Framework*, 0: 15.

———. 1994. *Teaching To Transgress* (Routledge: London).

———. 2016. 'Toward a Worldwide Culture of Love', retrieved 1 April 2016 from www.lionsroar.com/toward-a-worldwide-culture-of-love.

Horton, Carol. 2012. *Yoga Ph. D.: Integrating the Life of the Mind and the Wisdom of the Body* (Kleio Books: Chicago).

———. 2015. 'Yoga Selfies on Instagram: Reflections of a Curious Onlooker', retrieved 13 April 2015 from http://carolhortonphd.com/yoga-selfies-on-instagram.

———. 2016. 'Yoga 2016: Fragmented, Contested, Reimagined', retrieved 4 February 16 from http://yogadork.com/2016/01/19/yoga-2016-fragmented-contested-reimagined.

———. 2018. 'Reimagining Yoga', Yoga International, retrieved 13 March 2018 from https://yogainternational.com/article/view/reimagining-yoga-holistic-wellness-social-connection-spiritual-revitalizati.

Horton, Carol, and Roseanne Harvey. 2012. *21st Century Yoga: Culture, Politics, and Practice* (On Demand Publishing, LLC-Create Space: Berkeley).

Hoskins, Andrew. 2016. 'Memory Ecologies', *Memory Studies*, 9: 348–57.

Howard, Robert Glenn. 2013. 'Vernacular Authority: Critically Engaging "Tradition"', in Trevor J. Blank and Robert Glenn Howard (eds), *Tradition in the Twenty-First Century : Locating the Role of the Past in the Present* (Utah State University Press: Logan).

Hutchinson, Nick, and Anna Bodicoat. 2015. 'The Effectiveness of Intensive Interaction, A Systematic Literature Review', *Journal of Applied Research in Intellectual Disabilities*, 28: 437–54.

Ingold, Tim. 2011. *Being Alive: Essays on Movement, Knowledge and Description* (Routledge: London).

———. 2016. 'A Naturalist Abroad in the Museum of Ontology: Philippe Descola's Beyond Nature and Culture', *Anthropological Forum*, 26: 301–20.

Institute of Development Studies. 2009. 'Power Pack: Understanding Power for Social Change', unpublished work, University of Sussex.

IYN. 2018. 'School Membership', retrieved 16 January 2018 from https://independentyoganetwork.org/register/schools.

Jacobs, Stephen. 2017. 'Yoga Jam: Remixing kirtan in the Art of Living', *Journal of Religion and Popular Culture*, 29: 1–18.

Jacobs, Stephen, and Theo Wildcroft. 2017. 'Hindu Traditions in Contemporary British Communities', retrieved 4 June 2020 from www.religiousstudiesproject. com/podcast/hindu-traditions-in-contemporary-british-communities

Jain, Andrea R. 2012. 'Branding Yoga', *Approaching Religion*, 2: 3–15.

——. 2014a. *Selling Yoga: From Counterculture to Pop Culture* (Oxford University Press: Oxford).

——. 2014b. 'Who Is to Say Modern Yoga Practitioners Have It All Wrong? On Hindu Origins and Yogaphobia', *Journal of the American Academy of Religion*, 82: 427–71.

Jefferies, Luke. 2009. 'Introducing Intensive Interaction', *Psychologist*, 22: 756–58.

Jenkins, Henry, and Nico Carpentier. 2013. 'Theorizing Participatory Intensities: A Conversation about Participation and Politics', *Convergence*, 19: 265–86.

Jesson, Thomas. 2017. 'Upright and Uptight: The Invention of Posture', retrieved 10 April 2017 from https://medium.com/@thomas_jesson/upright-and-uptight-the-invention-of-posture-fe48282a4487.

Johnson, Don. 1997. 'Introduction', in Don Johnson (ed.), *Groundworks: Narratives of Embodiment* (North Atlantic Books: Berkeley, CA).

Johnson, Kimberley. 2011. 'Count Me Out of the Positivity Cult' from http://recoveringyogi.com/count-me-out-of-the-positivity-cult.

Johnson, Paul C. 2002. 'Migrating Bodies, Circulating Signs: Brazilian Candomble, the Garifuna of the Caribbean, and the Category of Indigenous Religions', *History of Religions*, 41: 301–27.

Johnson, Scott. 2018. 'Listen without Prejudice', retrieved 4 June 2018 from www.stillpointyogalondon.com/listen-without-prejudice.

Joldersma, Clarence W. 2013. 'Radical Constructivism, Education, and Truth as Life-Giving Disclosure', in L. Zuidervaart, A. Carr, M. Klaassen and R. Shuker (eds), *Truth Matters: Knowledge, Politics, Ethics, Religion.* (McGill-Queens Univ Press: Montreal), 46–65.

Jones, Suzanne E. 2017. *Mindful Touch: A Guide to Hands-On Support in Trauma-Sensitive Yoga* (Yoga Service Council: [Rhinebeck, NY?]).

Junker, Debora B. A. 2013. 'Zone of Proximal Development, Liminality, and Communitas: Implications for Religious Education', *Religious Education*, 108: 164–79.

Kaminoff, Leslie. 2018. 'I teach Viniyoga®. So, Sue Me', retrieved 13 March 2018 from www.yogaanatomy.org/so-sue-me.

Kane, Emily. 2018. 'Excessive Anatomy in Yoga Classes', retrieved 16 January 2018 from www.yogateachertrainingyogacara.com/excessive-anatomy-yoga-classes-yogacara-yoga-teacher-training.

Khouri, Hala. 2016. 'Trauma-Informed Yoga: Concepts, Tools, and Skills', unpublished manual

Knott, Kim. 2009. 'From Locality to Location and Back Again: A Spatial Journey in the Study of Religion', *Religion*, 39: 154–60.

Koch, Anne. 2015. 'Competitive Charity: A Neoliberal Culture of 'Giving Back' in Global Yoga', *Journal of Contemporary Religion*, 30: 73–88.

Kovach, Judith. 2002. 'The Body as the Ground of Religion, Science, and Self', *Zygon*, 37: 941–61.

Kraft, Siv-Ellen. 2002. '"To Mix or Not to Mix": Syncretism/Anti-syncretism in the History of Theosophy (A Discussion of the Innovative Contributions and Theoretical Relevance of Modern "Alternative" Religiosity)', *Numen-International Review for the History of Religions*, 49: 142–77.

Kramer, Joel, and Diana Alstad. 2012. *The Guru Papers: Masks of Authoritarian Power* (North Atlantic Books: Berkeley).

Kripal, Jeffrey J. 2001. 'One Lifetime, Many Lives: The Experience of Modern Hindu Hagiography', *History of Religions*, 40: 396–98.

Kripalu Center for Yoga & Health. 2017. 'Kripalu Yoga', retrieved 9 May 2017 from https://kripalu.org.

Krishna, TM. 2016. 'The Sri Sri Syndrome: What We Should Not Forget about so-called Gurus and Godmen', retrieved 4 April 2016 from http://scroll.in/article/805940/the-sri-sri-syndrome-what-we-should-not-forget-about-so-called-gurus-and-godmen.

LaBerge, Stephen. 1985. *Lucid Dreaming* (J.P. Tarcher: Los Angeles).

Lakoff, George, and Mark Johnson. 1999. *Philosophy in the Flesh : The Embodied Mind and its Challenge to Western Thought* (Basic Books: New York).

LaMothe, Kimerer L. 2008. 'What Bodies Know About Religion and the Study of It', *Journal of the American Academy of Religion*, 76: 573–601.

———. 2015. *Why we Dance : A Philosophy of Bodily Becoming* (Columbia University Press: New York).

Langford, Jean. 2004. *Fluent Bodies : Ayurvedic Remedies for Postcolonial Imbalance* (Oxford University Press: New York).

Langølen, Lars J. 2012. 'Yoga, Change and Embodied Enlightenment', *Approaching Religion*, 2: 27–37.

Latour, Bruno. 2004. 'How to Talk About the Body? The Normative Dimension of Science Studies', *Body & Society*, 10: 205–29.

Lavrence, Christine, and Kristin Lozanski. 2014. '"This Is Not Your Practice Life": Lululemon and the Neoliberal Governance of Self', *Canadian Review of Sociology/Revue canadienne de sociologie*, 51: 76–94.

Leach, John. 2016. 'Psychological Factors in Exceptional, Extreme and Torturous Environments', *Extreme Physiology & Medicine*, 5: 15.

Lederman, Eyal. 2010. 'The Fall of the Postural–Structural–Biomechanical Model in Manual and Physical Therapies: Exemplified by Lower Back Pain', *CPDO Online Journal*, March: 1–14.

Leledaki, Aspasia, and David Brown. 2009. '"Physicalisation": A Pedagogy of Body-Mind Cultivation for Liberation in Modern Yoga and Meditation Methods', *Asian Medicine*, 4: 303–37.

Levasseur, Barbie. 2015. '6 Steps For Success Every New Yoga Teacher Should Know', retrieved 11 April 2016 from www.myinnerfire.com/blogs/blog/42417857-6-steps-for-success-every-new-yoga-teacher-should-know.

Liberman, Kenneth. 2008. 'The Reflexivity of the Authenticity of Hatha Yoga', *Yoga in the Modern World: Contemporary Perspectives*: 100–16.

Lionel, Lesley, and Leonard Le Grange. 2011. 'Sustainability and Higher Education: From arborescent to rhizomatic thinking', *Educational Philosophy and Theory*, 43: 742–54.

Lipsius, David, and Theo Wildcroft. 2018. 'Theo Wildcroft: Complexities of Defining a Scope of Practice', in *Yoga Alliance*.

Lizardo, Omar. 2004. 'The Cognitive Origins of Bourdieu's Habitus', *Journal for the Theory of Social Behaviour*, 34: 375–401.

Long, Jeffery D. 2014. 'The Transformation of Yoga and Hinduism: Negotiating Authenticity, Innovation, and Identity in a Global Context', *Religious Studies Review*, 40: 125–32.

Longstaff, Jeffrey S. 1996. *Cognitive Structures of Kinaesthetic Space: Reevaluating Rudolf Laban's Choreutics in the Context of Spatial Cognition and Motor Control* (City University London and Laban Centre: London).

Lucas, Anneke. 2016. 'Why The Abused Don't Speak Up', retrieved 1 April 2014 from www.yogacitynyc.com/#!Why-The-Abused-Dont-Speak-Up/c1m6q/56d9acf40cf25a66a537df91.

Lussier-Ley, Chantale. 2010. 'Dialoguing with Body: A Self Study in Relational Pedagogy through Embodiment and the Therapeutic Relationship', *Qualitative Report*, 15: 197–214.

Lutz, Andrea. 2015. 'Ashtanga Yoga – The Asanas of the Primary Series', Ashtanga Studio Berlin, retrieved 12 August 2015. ashtangastudio.de/de/img/primaryserieschartA4_001.pdf.

Mallinson, James, and Mark Singleton. 2017. *Roots of Yoga* (Penguin Books: London).

Mantin, Ruth. 2004. 'Theological Reflections on Embodiment', *Feminist Theology: The Journal of the Britain & Ireland School of Feminist Theology*, 12: 212–27.

Maya, Kavita. 2015. 'Engendering Difference: The (Post)colonial Politics of Goddess Spirituality', conference paper, Utrecht University, retrieved 4 June 2020 from www.academia.edu/10889949/Engendering_Difference_The_Post_colonial_Politics_of_Goddess_Spirituality

McGuire, Meredith B. 1990. 'Religion and the Body: Rematerializing the Human Body in the Social Sciences of Religion', *Journal for the Scientific Study of Religion*, 29: 283.

McHose, Caryn, and Kevin Frank. 2006. *How Life Moves: Explorations in Meaning and Body Awareness* (North Atlantic Books: Berkeley).

McIlwain, Doris, and John Sutton. 2014. 'Yoga From the Mat Up: How Words Alight on Bodies', *Educational Philosophy and Theory*, 46: 655–73.

McKean, Lise. 1996. *Divine Enterprise: Gurus and the Hindu Nationalist Movement* (University of Chicago Press: Chicago).

Mellor, Philip A., and Chris Shilling. 2010. 'Body Pedagogics and the Religious Habitus: A New Direction for the Sociological Study of Religion', *Religion*, 40: 27–38.

Miles-Watson, Jonathan. 2016. 'Teachings of Tara: Sacred Place and Human Wellbeing in the Shimla Hills', *Anthropology in Action*, 23: 30–42.

Miller, Richard. 2010. *Yoga Nidra: A Meditative Practice for Deep Relaxation and Healing* (Sounds True: Louisville, KY).

Miller, Richard, and Eric Schoomaker. 2015. *The iRest Program for Healing PTSD : A Proven-Effective Approach to Using Yoga Nidra Meditation and Deep Relaxation Techniques to Overcome Trauma* (New Harbinger Publications: Oakland, CA).

Mitchell, Jules. 2014. 'You Aren't Tight, You Feel Tight', retrieved 9 July 2015 from www.julesmitchell.com/you-arent-tight-you-feel-tight.

Moberg, Marcus, and Tommy Ramstedt. 2016. 'Re-contextualizing the Framework of Scene for the Empirical Study of Post-institutional Religious Spaces in Practice', *Fieldwork in Religion*, 10: 155–72.

Moerman, Daniel E., and Wayne B. Jonas. 2002. 'Deconstructing the Placebo Effect and Finding the Meaning Response', *Annals of Internal Medicine*, 136: 471–76.

Mondada, Lorenza. 2012. 'Video Analysis and the Temporality of Inscriptions within Social Interaction: The Case of Architects at Work', *Qualitative Research*, 12: 304–33.

Moore, Candace. 2013. 'How to Do Supported Headstand', retrieved 16 January 2018 from www.yogabycandace.com/blog/2013/8/30/how-to-do-supported-headstand.

Mould, Oli. 2017. 'The Calais Jungle: A Slum of London's Making', *City*, 21: 388–404.

Mullan, Kelly Jean. 2014. 'Somatics: Investigating the Common Ground of Western Body–Mind Disciplines', *Body, Movement and Dance in Psychotherapy*, 9(4): 1–13.

Neitz, Mary Jo. 2013. 'Feminist Methodologies', in Michael Stausberg and Steven Engler (eds), *The Routledge Handbook of Research Methods in the Study of Religion* (Routledge: London).

Newcombe, Suzanne. 2009. 'The Development of Modern Yoga: A Survey of the Field', *Religion Compass*, 3.

——. 2011. 'Yoga in Modern Society', *Journal of Contemporary Religion*, 26: 518–19.

——. 2013. 'Magic and Yoga: The Role of Subcultures in Transcultural Exchange', in Beatrix Hauser (ed.), *Yoga Traveling: Bodily Practice in Transcultural Perspective* (Springer International Publishing: New York).

——. 2016. 'What is "Tradition"? Entanglements and Metaphors', retrieved 20 September 2016 from http://ayuryog.org/blog/what-%E2%80%98tradition%E2%80%99-%E2%80%93-entanglements-and-metaphors.

——. 2017. 'The Revival of Yoga in Contemporary India', retrieved 13 July 2017 from http://religion.oxfordre.com/view/10.1093/acrefore/97801993 40378.001.0001/acrefore-9780199340378-e-253?rskey=iBd83P&result=3.

NHS Fitness Studio. 2016. 'Vinyasa Flow Yoga Video', retrieved 6 January 2017 from www.nhs.uk/Conditions/nhs-fitness-studio/Pages/yoga-with-lj.aspx.

Nummenmaa, Lauri, Enrico Glerean, Mikko Viinikainen, Iiro P. Jaaskelainen, Rita Hari, and Mikko Sams. 2012. 'Emotions Promote Social Interaction by Synchronizing Brain Activity across Individuals', *Proceedings of the National Academy of Sciences of the United States of America*, 109: 9599–604.

Nye, Malory. 2000. 'Religion, Post-religionism, and Religioning: Religious Studies and Contemporary Cultural Debates', *Method and Theory in the Study of Religion*, 12: 447–76.

O'Sullivan, Jennifer. 2017. 'A Code of Ethics for Yoga Teachers ~ a Draft', retrieved 13 July 2017 from https://medium.com/@satiJen/code-of-ethics-for-yoga-teachers-a-draft-e96f0ce256f1.

Oh, Seil, and Natalia Sarkisian. 2012. 'Spiritual Individualism or Engaged Spirituality? Social Implications of Holistic Spirituality among Mind-Body-Spirit Practitioners', *Sociology of Religion*, 73: 299–322.

Olaveson, Tim. 2004. '"Connectedness" and the Rave Experience: Rave as New Religious Movement?', in Graham St John (ed.), *Rave Culture and Religion* (Routledge: London).

Orsi, Robert A. 2003. 'Is the Study of Lived Religion Irrelevant to the World we Live in? Special Presidential Plenary Address, Society for the Scientific Study of Religion, Salt Lake City, November 2, 2002', *Journal for the Scientific Study of Religion*, 42: 169–74.

——. 2012. 'Afterword: Everyday Religion and the Contemporary World', in Samuli Schielke and Liza Debevec (eds), *Ordinary Lives and Grand Schemes: An Anthropology of Everyday Religion* (Berghahn Books: Oxford).

——. 2013. 'Doing Religious Studies with Your Whole Body', *Practical Matters Journal*, 6.

Partridge, Christopher H. 2005. *The Re-enchantment of the West, Volume 2: Alternative Spiritualities, Sacralization, Popular Culture, and Occulture* (T&T Clark International: London).

Patankar, Prachi. 2014. 'Ghosts of Yogas Past and Present', retrieved 29 September 2016 from www.jadaliyya.com/pages/index/16632/ghosts-of-yogas-past-and-present.

Pettit, Andrew. 2014. 'Spiritual but not Religious: Understanding New Forms of Spirituality, Community, and Worship through the Musical Practice of Kirtan', *International Journal of Religion & Spirituality in Society*, 3: 13–18.

PlanC. 2015. 'We Are All Very Anxious', retrieved 4 April 2015 from www.weareplanc.org/blog/we-are-all-very-anxious.

Poole, Katy. 2012. 'The Vicious Vocal Minority vs. John Friend', retrieved 12 August 2015 from www.elephantjournal.com/2012/05/the-vicious-vocal-minority-vs-john-friend.

Powell, Seth. 2017. 'Advice on Āsana in the Śivayogapradīpikā', retrieved 13 July 2017 from http://theluminescent.blogspot.co.uk/2017/06/advice-on-asana-in-sivayogapradipika.html.

Preston, Stephanie D., and Frans B. M. de Waal. 2002. 'Empathy: Its Ultimate and Proximate Bases', *Behavioral and Brain Sciences*, 25: 1–71.

Primiano, Leonard N. 1995. 'Vernacular Religion and the Search for Method in Religious Folklife', *Western Folklore*, 54: 37–56.

Puustinen, Liina, and Matti Rautaniemi. 2015. 'Wellbeing for Sale: Representations of Yoga in Commercial Media', *Temenos*, 51: 45–70.

Pye, Michael. 2013. *Exploring Religions in Motion* (De Gruyter: Boston).

Rain, Karen. 2018. 'Yoga and #MeToo: Toward A Culture With Zero Tolerance For Sexual Assault', retrieved 29 January 2018 from www.decolonizingyoga.com/yoga-metoo-toward-culture-zero-tolerance-sexual-assault.

Rappaport, Roy A. 1999. *Ritual and Religion in the Making of Humanity* (Cambridge University Press: Cambridge).

Remski, Matthew. 2012. *Threads of Yoga: A Remix of Patanjalis Sutras, With Commentary and Reverie* (CreateSpace Independent Publishing Platform: Charleston).

——. 2014a. 'Boycott Satyananda's Literature and Methods Until Reparations are Made for Sexual Abuse', retrieved 15 December 2014 from http://matthewremski.com/wordpress/boycott-satyanandas-literature-and-methods-until-reparations-are-made-for-sexual-abuse.

——. 2014b. 'WAWADIA Update #18: One Hundred Years of Yoga in One Big Apple Day', retrieved 8 July 2015 from http://matthewremski.com/wordpress/wawadia-update-18-one-hundred-years-of-yoga-in-one-big-apple-day.

——. 2014c. 'WAWADIA Update #22: The Prescriptive Kinesiognomy of Modern Postural Yoga', retrieved 28 November 2014 from http://matthewremski.com/wordpress/wawadia-update-22-the-prescriptive-kinesiognomy-of-mpy.

——. 2014d. 'WAWADIA: A Prospectus', retrieved 7 November 2014 from www.indiegogo.com/projects/what-are-we-actually-doing-in-asana.

——. 2015a. 'Two Wings of Yogic Self-Care: Data and Intention (or Herbs and Sugar Pills)', retrieved 13 November 2015 from http://matthewremski.com/wordpress/two-wings-of-yogic-self-care-data-and-intention-or-herbs-and-sugar-pills.

——. 2015b. 'WAWADIA Online Workshop', retrieved from www.mettaversity.com/what-are-we-actually-doing-in-asana-online-workshop.

——. 2015c. 'Yogapillgate: Discourse, Transparency, Epistemology, Magic', retrieved from http://matthewremski.com/wordpress/yogapillgate-discourse-transparency-epistemology-magic.

——. 2016a. 'Yoga Can Injure You. Here's How to Find a Class that Won't', retrieved 28 November 2016 from www.theguardian.com/commentisfree/

2016/oct/27/yoga-injury-class-regulation-bad-practitioners?CMP=share_btn_fb.

——. 2016b. 'Silence and Silencing at Jivamukti Yoga and Beyond', Be Scofield, retrieved 27 June 2016 from www.decolonizingyoga.com/silence-silencing-jivamukti-yoga-beyond.

——. 2017. 'Shadow Pose: A Secret History of Trauma and Healing in Modern Yoga', retrieved 4 August 2018 from www.facebook.com/matthewremski author/posts/the-book-that-has-evolved/1823649774592155.

——. 2018a. '"Feminist-Informed" Ashtanga and "Trauma-Informed" Kundalini: How Cultic Deception Can Harm Academics and Therapists', retrieved 20 November 2018 from http://matthewremski.com/wordpress/feminist-informed-ashtanga-and-trauma-informed-kundalini-how-cultic-deception-can-harm-academics-and-therapists/?fbclid=IwAR0Oho EQ4jECbxWcOj8A3In8nXhsKwaF_Yw0VWayKARMmvlOItVsyz0Zw-E.

——. 2018b. 'Yoga's Culture of Sexual Abuse: Nine Women Tell Their Stories', retrieved 4 June 2018 from https://thewalrus.ca/yogas-culture-of-sexual-abuse-nine-women-tell-their-stories.

——. 2019. *Practice and All Is Coming: Abuse, Cult Dynamics, and Healing in Yoga and Beyond* (Embodied Wisdom Publishing: Kentucky).

Reymond, Lizelle. 1985. *The Dedicated: A Biography of Nivedita* (Samata Books: Madras).

Reynolds, Kathleen. 2015. '"Who's Flying this Plane?" The Blind Leading the Blind in Western Yoga', retrieved 1 April 2016 from www.hinduhumanrights.info/whos-flying-this-plane-the-blind-leading-the-blind-in-western-yoga.

Ridout, Nicholas. 2008. 'Performance and Democracy', in Tracey C Davis (ed.), *The Cambridge Companion to Performance Studies* (Cambridge University Press: Cambridge).

Robertson, Alison, and Theo Wildcroft. 2017. 'Sacrifices at the Altar of Self-transformation', *Body and Religion*, 1: 88–109.

Robson, Colin. 2002. *Real World Research: A Resource for Social Scientists and Practitioner-Researchers* (Wiley-Blackwell: Oxford).

Rosa, Hartmut. 2004. 'Four Levels of Self-interpretation', *Philosophy & Social Criticism*, 30: 691–720.

Rowe, James K. 2015. 'Zen and the Art of Social Movement Maintenance', retrieved 21/3/2015 from http://wagingnonviolence.org/feature/mindfulness-and-the-art-of-social-movement-maintenance.

Royal Academy of Dance. 2014. 'The Benesh Movement Notation Score', retrieved 30 December 2014 from www.rad.org.uk/documents/benesh-docs/benesh-movement-notation-score-updated-nov2014.pdf.

Ruiz, Fernando P. 2007. 'The Sticky Business + History of Yoga Mats', retrieved 24 March 2018 from www.yogajournal.com/yoga-101/sticky-business.

Sabatini, Sandra, and Jan Heron. 2006. *Breath: The Essence of Yoga* (Pinter & Martin: London).

Samaj, Haidakhandi. 2017. 'Babaji', retrieved 9 May 2017 from www.haidak handisamaj.org/babaji.

Sanders, Joshunda, and Ana Mouyis. 2010. 'Eat, Pray, Spend: Priv-lit and the New, Enlightened American Dream', retrieved 16 October 2015 from https:// bitchmedia.org/article/eat-pray-spend.

Santosa. 2014. 'A Taste of Santosa', retrieved 4 June 2020 from www.youtube. com/watch?v=p6TO3f8p0PM.

Saraswati, Swami Satyananda. 2013. *Asana, Pranayama, Mudra, Bandha* (Yoga Publications Trust: Bihar).

Sarbacker, Stuart R. 2014. 'Reclaiming the Spirit through the Body: The Nascent Spirituality of Modern Postural Yoga', *Entangled Religions*, 1: 95–114.

Savage, Mike, Fiona Devine, Niall Cunningham, Mike Taylor, Yaojun J. Li, Johs Hjellbrekke, Brigitte Le Roux, Sam Friedman, and Andrew Miles. 2013. 'A New Model of Social Class? Findings from the BBC's Great British Class Survey Experiment', *Sociology: the Journal of the British Sociological Association*, 47: 219–50.

Scaravelli, Vanda. 1991. *Awakening the Spine* (HarperCollins: New York).

Schnabele, Verena. 2013. 'The Useful Body: The Yogic Answer to Appearance Management in the Post-Fordist', in Beatrix Hauser (ed.), *Yoga Traveling: Bodily Practice in Transcultural Perspective* (Springer International Publishing: New York).

Schuler, Sabastian. 2011. 'Synchronized Ritual Behavior: Religion, Cognition and the Dynamics of Embodiment', in David Cave and Rebecca S. Norris (eds), *Religion and the Body: Modern Science and the Construction of Religious Meaning* (Brill: Boston).

Scofield, Be. 2018. 'The Yoga Barn Guru: Inside Uma Inder's Bali Cult', retrieved 14 May 2018 from https://medium.com/@bescofield/the-yoga-barn-guru- inside-uma-inders-bali-cult-6ac69cdc678b.

Sewell, William H. 1992. 'A Theory of Structure: Duality, Agency, and Trans- formation', *American Journal of Sociology*, 98: 1–29.

Shaw, Hollie. 2018. 'Yoga Apparel Maker Lululemon's Fourth-Quarter Sales, Profits Surge', Financial Post, retrieved 14 May 2018 from http://business.financial post.com/news/retail-marketing/yoga-apparel-maker-lululemons- fourth-quarter-sales-profits-surge.

Shearer, Alistair. 2010. *The Yoga Sutras of Patanjali* (Bell Tower: New York).

Sheets-Johnstone, Maxine. 2007. 'Consciousness: A Natural History', *Synthesis Philosophica*, 22: 283–99.

——. 2009. 'Animation: The Fundamental, Essential, and Properly Descriptive Concept', *Continental Philosophy Review*, 42: 375–400.

——. 2010. 'Somatic Perspectives on Psychotherapy', retrieved 4 June 2020 from somaticperspectives.com/2010/05/sheets-johnstone.

——. 2011. *The Primacy of Movement* (John Benjamins: Amsterdam).

——. 2012. 'Movement and Mirror Neurons: A Challenging and Choice Conversation', *Phenomenology and the Cognitive Sciences*, 11: 385–401.

———. 2017. 'Moving in Concert', *Choros International Dance Journal*, 6: 1–19.

Shor, Ira. 2002. 'Education is Politics: Paulo Freire's Critical Pedagogy', in Peter Leonard and Peter McLaren (eds), *Paulo Freire: A Critical Encounter* (Routledge: London).

Simpkin, Arabella L., and Richard M. Schwartzstein. 2016. 'Tolerating Uncertainty – The Next Medical Revolution?', *New England Journal of Medicine*, 375: 1713–15.

Singleton, Mark. 2010. *Yoga Body: The Origins of Modern Posture Practice* (Oxford University Press: Oxford).

———. 2013. 'Transnational Exchange and the Genesis of Modern Postural Yoga', in Beatrix Hauser (ed.), *Yoga Traveling: Bodily Practice in Transcultural Perspective* (Springer International Publishing: New York).

Singleton, Mark, and Jean Byrne. 2008. *Yoga in the Modern World: Contemporary Perspectives* (Routledge: London).

Singleton, Mark, and Ellen Goldberg. 2013a. *Gurus of Modern Yoga* (Oxford University Press: Oxford).

———. 2013b. 'Introduction', in Mark Singleton and Ellen Goldberg (eds), *Gurus of Modern Yoga* (Oxford University Press: Oxford).

SkillsActive. 2017. 'Yoga NOS – FAQs', retrieved 21 January 2018 from www.skillsactive.com/faqs.

Slee, Roger, Andrew Azzopardi, and Shaun Grech. 2012. *Inclusive Communities: A Critical Reader* (Sense Publishers: Rotterdam).

Smith, Bejamin R. 2008. '"With Heat Even Iron Will Bend": Discipline and Authority in Ashtanga Yoga', in Mark Singleton and Jean Byrne (eds), *Yoga in the Modern World Contemporary Perspectives* (Routledge: London).

Smith, Sarai Harvey. 2018. 'The Sexual Misconduct of Pattabhi Jois: My Thoughts, Accountability, and 5 Changes to Pledge my Support for the Victims', retrieved 4 June 2018 from https://saraiyoga.wordpress.com/2018/03/17/the-sexual-misconduct-of-pattabhi-jois-my-thoughts-accountability-and-5-changes-to-pledge-my-support-for-the-victims.

Sparkes, Andrew C., and Brett Smith. 2011. 'Inhabiting Different Bodies over Time: Narrative and Pedagogical Challenges', *Sport, Education and Society*, 16: 357–70.

Spickard, James V. 2005. 'Ritual, Symbol, and Experience: Understanding Catholic Worker House Masses', *Sociology of Religion*, 66: 337–57.

Spivak, Gayatri C. 2008. 'Can the Subaltern Speak?' in Joanne Sharp (ed.), *Geographies of Postcolonialism* (Sage Publications: Thousand Oaks).

Spretnak, Charlene. 2012. *The Resurgence of the Real: Body, Nature and Place in a Hypermodern World* (Routledge: London).

Standing, Guy. 2011. *The Precariat: The New Dangerous Class* (Bloomsbury Publishing: London).

Steinberg, Deborah Lynn, and Margrit Shildrick. 2015. 'Estranged Bodies: Shifting Paradigms and the Biomedical Imaginary', *Body & Society*, 21: 3–19.

Stirk, John. 2015. *The Original Body: Deepening Practice for the Teaching of Yoga* (Handspring Publishing: Edinburgh).

Storr, Anthony. 1997. *Feet Of Clay* (Free Press: New York).

Strauss, Sarah, and Laura Mandelbaum. 2013. 'Discourses on Sustainable Living', in Beatrix Hauser (ed.), *Yoga Traveling: Bodily Practice in Transcultural Perspective* (Springer International Publishing: New York).

Sullivan, Marlysa B., Matt Erb, Laura Schmalzl, Steffany Moonaz, Jessica Noggle Taylor, and Stephen W. Porges. 2018. 'Yoga Therapy and Polyvagal Theory: The Convergence of Traditional Wisdom and Contemporary Neuroscience for Self-Regulation and Resilience.(Report)', *Frontiers in Human Neuroscience*, 12.

Sutton, John. 2011. 'Influences on Memory', *Memory Studies*, 4: 355–59.

Sweetman, Paul. 2013. 'Structure, Agency, Subculture: The CCCS, Resistance through Rituals, and 'Post-Subcultural' Studies', *Sociological Research Online*, 18: 10.

Takahashi, Melanie. 2004. 'The "Natural High": Altered States, Flashbacks and Neural Tuning at Raves', in Graham St John (ed.), *Rave Culture and Religion* (Routledge: London).

Taylor, Mary. 2018. '#TimesUp: Ending Sexual Abuse in the Yoga Community', retrieved 24 March 2018 from www.yogajournal.com/lifestyle/timesup-metoo-ending-sexual-abuse-in-the-yoga-community.

Thompson, Becky, and Rolf Gates. 2014. *Survivors on the Yoga Mat: Stories for Those Healing from Trauma* (North Atlantic Books: Berkeley).

Thoreau, Henry D. 2003. *A Week on the Concord and Merrimack Rivers* (Project Gutenberg: Gutenberg.org).

Tredwell, Gail. 2013. *Holy Hell: A Memoir of Faith, Devotion, and Pure Madness* (BookBaby: Oregon).

Tuck-Po, Lye. 2008. 'Before a Step Too Far: Walking with Batek Hunter-Gatherers in the Forests of Pahang, Malaysia', in Tim and Vergunst Ingold, Jo Lee (ed.), *Ways of Walking* (Ashgate: Aldershot).

Tumminello, Nick, and Jason Silvernail. 2017. 'The Corrective Exercise Trap', retrieved 11 June 2017 from www.nsca.com/Pages/ContentRightNav.aspx?pageid=36507234762.

Tweed, Thomas A. 2006. *Crossing and Dwelling : A Theory of Religion* (Harvard University Press: Cambridge, MA).

Ulland, Dagfinn. 2012. 'Embodied Spirituality', *Archive for the Psychology of Religion-Archiv Fur Religionspsychologie*, 34: 83–104.

Urban, Hugh B. 2000. 'The Cult of Ecstasy: Tantrism, the New-Age, and the Spiritual Logic of Late Capitalism (Interpreting Eastern Philosophies in a "Late Capitalist" World Order of Pluralism and Globalism)', *History of Religions*, 39: 268–304.

——. 2004. 'Magia Sexualis: Sex, Secrecy, and Liberation in Modern Western Esotericism', *Journal of the American Academy of Religion*, 72: 695–731.

Van der Kolk, Bessel A. 2014. *The Body Keeps the Score: Mind, Brain and Body in the Transformation of Trauma* (Allen Lane: London).

Van der Zee, Hendrik. 1996. 'The Learning Society: Challenges and Trends', in R et al Edwards (ed.), *The Learning Society: Challenges and Trends* (Routledge: London).

van Kooten, Victor. 1997. *From Inside Out: A Yoga Notebook from the Teachings of Angela & Victor* (Sequoyah Graphics: Oakland).

van Loon, Joost. 2006. 'Network', *Theory Culture & Society*, 23: 307–14.

Venkatesan, Archana. 2014. 'Making Saints, Making Communities: Nayaki Svamikal and the Saurashtras of Madurai', *South Asia-Journal of South Asian Studies*, 37: 568–85.

Vitalis, Daniel. 2016. 'Are you Kinaesthetically Literate? – Tom Myers #101', retrieved 4 June 2020 from www.danielvitalis.com/rewild-yourself-podcast/ are-you-kinesthetically-literate-tom-myers-101.

Viveiros de Castro, Eduardo. 2014. 'Who is Afraid of the Ontological Wolf?' CUSAS Annual Marilyn Strathern Lecture, Cambridge, 30 May.

Voelkl, B., and J. Fritz. 2017. 'Relation between Travel Strategy and Social Organization of Migrating Birds with Special Consideration of Formation Flight in the Northern Bald Ibis', *Philosophical Transactions of the Royal Society B-Biological Sciences*, 372: 11.

Wacquant, Loic. 2014. 'Homines in Extremis: What Fighting Scholars Teach Us about Habitus', *Body & Society*, 20: 3–17.

Walford, Edward. 1878. 'Mayfair', British History Online from www.british-history.ac.uk/old-new-london/vol4/pp345-359.

Walker, Julian. 2012. 'Enlightenment 2.0: The American Yoga Experiment', in Carol Horton (ed.), *21st Century Yoga: Culture, Politics, and Practice* (Create Space: Berkeley).

Warrier, Maya. 2003. 'Processes of Secularization in Contemporary India: Guru Faith in the Mata Amritanandamayi Mission', *Modern Asian Studies*, 37: 213–53.

Wenger, Etienne. 1999. 'Community', in Etienne Wenger (ed.), *Communities of Practice: Learning, Meaning, and Identity* (Cambridge University Press: Cambridge).

Westoby, Ruth. 2018. 'The Esoteric Feminine In Hathayoga Sources', in *Embodied Philosophy Yoga Reconsidered: Modern Yoga Research*, edited by Jacob Kyle, retrieved from http://embodiedphilosophy.courses.

Wharton, Amy S. 2009. 'The Sociology of Emotional Labor', *Annual Review of Sociology*, 35: 147–65.

White, David G. 1984. 'Why Gurus are Heavy', *Numen*, 31: 40–73.

White, David Gordon. 2006. '"Open" and "Closed" Models of the Human Body In Indian Medical and Yogic Traditions', *Asian Medicine*, 2: 1–13.

White, Micah. 2016. *The End of Protest : A New Playbook for Revolution* (Alfred A. Knopf Canada: Toronto).

Whitehead, Amy. 2008. 'The Goddess and the Virgin: Materiality in Western Europe', *Pomegranate*, 10: 163–83.

Wilson, Margaret. 2002. 'Six Views of Embodied Cognition', *Psychonomic Bulletin & Review*, 9: 625–36.

Wittel, Andreas. 2001. 'Toward a Network Sociality', *Theory Culture & Society*, 18: 51–76.

Worthington, Andy. 2004. *Stonehenge: Celebration and Subversion* (Alternative Albion: Loughborough).

Wujastyk, Dagmar. 2017. 'How to Respond to Yogic Powers', retrieved 19 November 2017 from http://ayuryog.org/blog/how-respond-yogic-powers.

Wujastyk, Dominik. 2011. 'Medical Error and Medical Truth: The Placebo Effect and Room for Choice in Ayurveda', *Health, Culture and Society*, 1: 222–31.

Wulf, Gabriele. 2013. 'Attentional Focus and Motor Learning: A Review of 15 years', *International Review of Sport and Exercise Psychology*, 6: 77–104.

Yates, Pete. 2016. 'Response to NOS by IYN Secretary', retrieved 28 November 2016 from http://bgi.uk.com/2016/10/17/response-nos-iyn-secretary.

Yeats, William B. 1938. *The Ten Principal Upanishads* (Faber & Faber: London).

Yoga Alliance UK. 2016. 'Our VIEW – National Occupational Standards for Yoga', Yoga Alliance Professionals, retrieved 28 November 2016 from https://yogaalliance.co.uk/2016/10/28/our-view-national-occupational-standards-for-yoga.

Yoga Alliance UK. 2018. 'Yoga Alliance: Standards Review Project', retrieved 13 March 2018 from https://yastandards.com.

YogaDork. 2009. 'Yoga Teacher FAIL … Is that Pattabhi Jois? [photo]', retrieved 1 April 2016 from http://yogadork.com/2009/09/14/yoga-teacher-failis-that-pattabhi-jois-photo.

——. 2014. 'YogaDork Giveaway: Win a Print of The Yoga Poster – A Visual Map of Yoga's History', retrieved 29 January 2018 from http://yogadork.com/2014/12/22/yogadork-giveaway-win-a-print-of-the-yoga-poster-a-visual-map-of-yogas-history.

yogagurusrevealed. 2014. 'Pattabhi Jois: Ashtanga Yoga Adjustments', retrieved from decolonizingyoga.com.

Zimbler, Nicole. 2017. 'Yoga 4 Autism', retrieved 9 May 2017 from http://yoga4autism.org.

INDEX

www.ingramcontent.com/pod-product-compliance
Lightning Source LLC
Chambersburg PA
CBHW040145270326
41929CB00024B/3371